Healthy Kidney Cookbook: Nourishing Renal Recipes

Osama .D Lin

All rights reserved.

Copyright © 2024 Osama .D Lin

Healthy Kidney Cookbook: Nourishing Renal Recipes : Delicious and Nutritious Recipes for Optimal Kidney Health - Improve Your Well-being with Renal-friendly Meals!

Funny helpful tips:

Life's melody is ever-changing; tune in to its rhythm and harmonize with its beat.

Diversify your reading list; exposing yourself to various genres and cultures broadens your perspective.

Life advices:

Rotate between different subjects; it prevents cognitive fatigue and keeps the reading experience fresh.

Nurture your mental health; it's as crucial as physical well-being.

Introduction

Embark on a journey to support kidney health with this book, a comprehensive guide that combines nutritional knowledge with delicious recipes to help you navigate the challenges of kidney disease.

This cookbook begins with an overview of kidney disease, shedding light on how kidneys function, the types of kidney diseases, and the roots of kidney failure. Explore the symptoms, stages, and identification of chronic kidney disease, gaining insights into its management and prevention.

Dive into the heart of the renal diet, understanding its principles, and discovering the foods to include and omit for optimal kidney health. Uncover cooking tips specifically tailored to renal diets and find answers to the most common questions related to kidney health.

The cookbook then transforms knowledge into action, offering a variety of recipes to support a renal diet. From nourishing breakfast options to vibrant salads and soups, explore vegetarian and vegan entrées, snacks, condiments, and a diverse array of dishes featuring meat, poultry, fish, and seafood. Quench your thirst with beverages and smoothies, and satisfy your sweet tooth with delightful dessert recipes.

Whether you're navigating kidney disease or proactively supporting kidney health, this cookbook is your ally in creating flavorful, kidney-friendly meals. May your culinary journey be filled with nourishing dishes that contribute to the well-being of your kidneys and your overall health. Happy cooking!

Contents

Chapter 1:   Overview Of KidneyDisease 1

  1.1   How do your kidneys function? 2

  1.2   Kidney disease types.. 2

  1.3   The Roots of Kidney Failure... 3

  1.4   Symptoms and signs 4

  1.5   When does chronic kidney disease becomedangerous? 5

  1.6   Can chronic renal disease be classified intostages?.................. 6

  1.7   How to identify kidney disease?... 7

  1.8   Can Kidney Disease Be Cured? 7

  1.9   Can renal illness be prevented?... 8

Chapter 2:   The Renal Diet 10

  2.1   Renal diet: what is it? 10

  2.2   Foods to include in a renal diet 11

  2.3   Foods to omit from a renal diet 13

  2.5   Cooking tips for renal diets.. 16

  2.6   Most common questions 17

Chapter 3:   Breakfast recipes for arenal diet 20

  3.1   Scrambled eggs with cheese and fresh herbs 20

  3.2   Loaded Vegetable Eggs 21

  3.3   Chai apple smoothie... 22

  3.5   Breakfast green soup 24

  3.6   Apple-mint French toast 24

  3.7   Hot multigrain cereal.. 25

  3.8   Morning herb rolls 26

3.9 Buckwheat pancakes..27

3.10 Leek and Brussels sprout quiche...28

3.11 Chia pudding..30

3.12 Mexican breakfast eggs on toast...31

3.13 Stuffed omelet with vegetables..32

3.14 Breakfast burrito with green chilies..33

3.15 Blueberry pancakes...34

3.16 Egg and avocado bake...35

3.17 Broccoli-basil quiche..36

3.18 Asparagus frittata...37

3.20 Breakfast wrap with fruit and cheese..39

Chapter 4: Salads and Soups...41

4.1 Beef barley soup with vegetables...41

4.5 Pumpkin soup..46

4.6 A butternut squash soup..48

4.7 Red pepper roasted soup..49

4.10 Cauliflower curried soup...53

4.11 Watercress cream soup..54

4.12 Salad with strawberries and watercress withalmond dressing..................56

4.13 Lettuce salad with asparagus and raspberries................................57

4.14 Beef ginger salad..58

4.15 Confetti farfalle salad..60

4.16 Lemon-dressed cucumber-dill salad withcabbage...............................61

4.17 Chinese-style turkey salad...62

4.18 Watercress and pear salad..63

4.19 Salad of roasted beets...64

4.20 Arugula and celery salad...65

Chapter 5: Vegetarian and vegan entrées 67

    5.1   Spicy broccoli and tofu stir-fry 67

    5.2   Rice and collard-filled red peppers 68

    5.3   Vegan white bean burgers 70

    5.4   Strata of red peppers 71

    5.5   Thai-inspired vegetable curry 73

    5.6   Linguine with roasted red pepper–basil sauce 75

    5.7   Mie Goreng with broccoli 76

    5.8   Fried rice with vegetables 77

    5.9   Penne and egg white frittata 79

    5.10   Stuffed spaghetti squash with bulgur 80

    5.11   Egg and kale on bread 82

    5.12   Mac and cheese 83

    5.13   Eggplant and tofu stir-fry 85

    5.14   Vegetable Biryani 86

    5.15   Pesto cream pasta 88

    5.16   Bowl of roasted vegetables and barley 89

    5.17   Bulgur and vegetables loaded delicata squashboats 90

    5.18   Falafel spinach wrap 92

    5.19   Potato and cauliflower curry 93

    5.20   Sweet pepper, onion, and cabbage medley 94

Chapter 6: Snacks, condiments, and 96

    6.1   Delicious popcorn 96

    6.2   Raspberry cream nibbles 97

    6.4   Spicy and sweet kettle corn 99

    6.5   Tortilla chips flavored with cinnamon 100

    6.6   Meringue cookies 101

6.8	Red pepper crostini with chicken	103
6.10	Cheesy pineapple ball	105
6.11	Roasted mint-flavored carrots	106
6.12	Lime cilantro vinaigrette	107
6.13	Balsamic vinaigrette	108
6.14	Lime blueberry sauce	108
6.15	Cranberry cabbage	109

Chapter 7: Recipes for meat and poultry 111

7.1	Thai curried chicken	111
7.2	Aromatic chicken and cabbage stir-fry	112
7.3	Baked chicken with herbs	114
7.4	Sour and sweet meatloaf	115
7.5	Cucumber-cilantro salsa with grilled steak	116
7.6	Meatloaf with gravy from mushrooms	117
7.8	Asian-style chicken satay	120
7.9	Fettuccine with pork ragu	121

Chapter 8: Fish and seafood dishes 125

8.1	Garlic lemon halibut	125
8.2	Shrimp scampi linguine	126
8.3	Seafood casserole	127
8.4	Haddock baked in an herb crust	129
8.6	Fish with pineapple salsa	131
8.7	Kale and Salmon on parchment	132
8.8	Cod with dill - cucumber salsa	133
8.9	Grilled shrimp with a lime cucumber salsa	135
8.10	Linguine with scampi shrimp	136

Chapter 9: Beverages and smoothies 138

9.1 Berry-bursting smoothie 138

9.2 Berries mint water 139

9.3 Chia vanilla smoothie 139

9.4 Pina colada Smoothie 140

9.5 Oat banana shake 141

9.6 Smoothie with strawberry cheesecake 142

9.7 Apple lemon smoothie 143

9.8 Raspberry peach smoothie 143

9.10 Cinnamon horchata 145

9.11 Kiwi watermelon smoothie 146

9.12 Digestive cooler fennel 147

9.13 Cranberry and ginger punch 147

9.14 Orange and blueberry-infused water 148

9.15 Spinach and cucumber smoothie 149

Chapter 10: Desserts 151

10.1 Flavorful shortbread cookies 151

10.2 Tropical granita 152

10.3 Apple Dutch pancake 153

10.5 Raspberry mousse cheesecake 155

10.6 Meringue almond cookies 156

10.7 Peachy pavlova 157

10.8 Pecan and raisin cookies (without sugar) 159

10.9 Cinnamon custard 160

10.10   Pound cake (Low sodium) 161

Chapter 1: Overview Of Kidney Disease

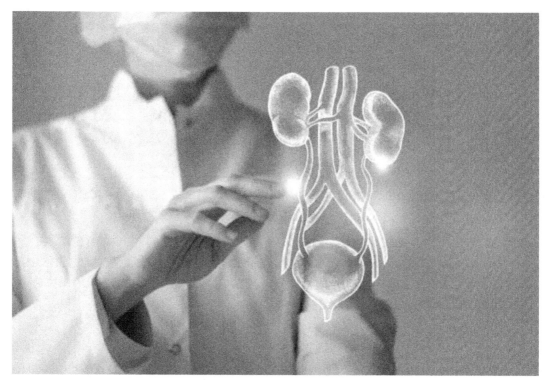

According to estimates, 31 million Americans alone are thought to be affected by renal disease, and 1 in 10 individuals worldwide suffer from it in some capacity. Kidney disease, often known as renal disease, is the umbrella term describing kidney diseases that impair function.

Kidney disease is characterized by damage to the kidneys, which prevents them from functioning optimally. Because kidney function gradually deteriorates over time, kidney disease is referred to as "chronic." Renal failure, often known as end-stage kidney disease, is the result of kidney disease. You will need dialysis (artificial filtration) or a kidney transplant at this point.

1.1 How do your kidneys function?

Kidneys are two in one. They are (bean-shaped) organs that are situated towards the base of the rib cage, along either side of the spine. The size of each kidney is around that of your fist.

Your kidneys filter your blood, eliminating pollutants, water, and salt, as urine. Waste products in the blood can be harmful if the kidneys aren't filtering them out properly due to injury or illness.

Additionally, your kidneys regulate the number of minerals and salts in your body, produce the hormones that regulate blood pressure, create red blood cells, and maintain the strength of your bones.

1.2 Kidney disease types

There are two basic categories of kidney illness: acute kidney injury and chronic kidney disease (chronic).

Acute renal injury and chronic kidney disease are the two main kinds of kidney disease (chronic kidney disease). Acute kidney disease usually resolves completely, but it can raise a person's chance of later-life chronic kidney disease.

1. Acute kidney disease

Acute renal injury refers to kidney damage that doesn't continue longer than three months. It often develops quickly in reaction to a kidney-related injury, disease, drug use, kidney obstructions, or a variety of other reasons. Some individuals will require a brief course of dialysis for their kidneys to heal.

Many people experience acute kidney injury, fully recover, and resume their regular lives. However, there is an increased chance of later developing chronic (or continuous) renal disease if major damage has already been done.

As a result, those who have experienced acute kidney injury must take extra care to track their kidney function permanently. One method to achieve this is to maintain healthy food and nutritional routine. Additionally, your doctor should assess the health of your kidneys every two years.

2. Chronic kidney disease

When your kidneys have sustained irreversible damage, chronic kidney disease results. The ailment must have existed for at least 3 months to be identified as chronic kidney disease.

Even with chronic renal disease, you can function normally for many years. However, a lot of patients will eventually require kidney replacement therapy as their kidneys' capacity to filter their blood continues to deteriorate. This could take the form of kidney transplantation or dialysis.

Chronic kidney disease has a wide range of potential causes, including genetics, infection, and immunological conditions that harm your kidneys.

If you have renal disease or another illness affecting the kidneys, it's important that you get a thorough explanation from your doctor about the specific sort of kidney disease or condition you have, what developed it, the best way to care for your kidneys, and how this will affect your daily life.

You are better able to control and possibly slow down the evolution of your ailment the more information you have.

1.3 <u>The Roots of Kidney Failure</u>

The inability of damaged kidneys to perform their normal function of filtering the blood leads to renal disease. When an accident or toxin is the source, the damage can occur immediately, but more often, it takes months or years to develop.

Diabetes and elevated blood pressure (hypertension) are the two main risk factors for chronic kidney disease. Various other illnesses and disorders can also impair kidney function and result in chronic renal disease:

- ◦ Glomerulonephritis. The filtration units of your kidneys, called glomeruli, are damaged in this condition.
- ◦ Polycystic renal disease. This genetic condition results in the development of several fluid-filled cysts in your kidneys, which impairs the kidneys' capacity to operate.
- ◦ Hypertensive nephrosclerosis. Chronic high blood pressure might be harmful to the kidneys.
- ◦ Membranous nephropathy. The immune system of your body targets the kidney's waste-filtering membranes in this condition.
- ◦ Kidney stones, a swollen prostate, or cancer can all obstruct the urinary tract.
- ◦ Vesicoureteral reflux. This condition causes the ureters to reabsorb urine, which then flows back up to the kidneys.
- ◦ Nephrotic syndrome. This is a combination of symptoms indicating renal impairment.
- ◦ Persistent kidney infection (pyelonephritis).
- ◦ Diabetes-related kidney damage. Numbness, tingling, muscle weakness, and pain are common symptoms of this type of injury or malfunction of one or more nerves brought on by diabetes.
- ◦ Lupus and some other immune system disorders, such as polyarteritis nodosa, Goodpasture syndrome, sarcoidosis, and Henoch-Schonlein purpura, affect the kidneys.

1.4 **Symptoms and signs**

You typically don't have any visible symptoms when the kidney disease is first developing. Indicators that the illness is progressing include:

A strong urge to urinate (pee).

- Your pee is frothy and contains blood.
- Decrease in appetite.
- Weakness, lack of energy, and weariness.
- Difficulty sleeping
- Elevated blood pressure
- Respiration difficulty.
- Your hands, ankles, and feet are swelling.
- Swollen eyes.
- Itchy and dry skin
- Having trouble focusing
- Numbness.
- Muscle pain.
- Sickness or vomiting
- A skin-color changes

Kidney disease symptoms and signs are frequently vague. They can, therefore, also be brought on by different diseases. You might not exhibit symptoms until irreparable harm has been done since your kidneys can compensate for reduced function.

1.5 <u>When does chronic kidney disease become dangerous?</u>

Your entire body will not function properly if your kidneys aren't functioning properly. Chronic renal disease has several side effects, including:

- Low level of red blood cells (anemia).
- Weak bones.
- Gout.
- Your risk of infection rises due to a decreased immune response.

- Metabolic acidosis. Your blood's chemical balance (acid-base imbalance) has changed because of decreased kidney function.
- Heart disease increases the risk of heart attack and stroke.
- High potassium levels (hyperkalemia) impair the proper operation of your heart.
- Fertility issues and erectile dysfunction.
- A lot of phosphorus (hyperphosphatemia).
- Elevated blood pressure
- Fluid accumulation can cause swelling in the hands, ankles, and feet, as well as in the lungs.

1.6 <u>Can chronic renal disease be classified into stages?</u>

A guideline was developed by the NKF (National Kidney Foundation) to assist physicians in determining the severity of kidney disease. Kidney disease (CKD) has five stages, according to the NKF.

Since each stage of kidney illness necessitates a particular course of therapy, knowing what stage a patient is in enables medical professionals to offer the best care.

We must first comprehend the measurement of kidney function to comprehend each step. Glomerular Filtration Rate is the generally accepted indicator of kidney function (GFR). How well your kidneys clear your blood is a measure of renal function.

The blood test to measure the amount of serum creatinine or the creatinine found in the blood—is the primary method of measuring GFR. Creatinine levels rise when renal function decreases.

The GFR is calculated using an equation. Along with serum creatinine, the equation also takes into account age, race, and gender. Blood urea nitrogen (BUN), weight, and serum albumin are additional variables that could be taken into consideration.

The 5 stages of kidney disease are depicted here, along with the GFR for each stage:

- In Stage 1: (GFR > 90 mL/min) with high or normal GFR
- In Stage 2: (GFR = 60-89 mL/min) Mild CKD
- In Stage 3(A): (GFR = 45-59 mL/min) Moderate CKD
- In Stage 3(B): (GFR = 30-44 mL/min) Moderate CKD
- In Stage 4: (GFR = 15-29 mL/min) Severe CKD
- In Stage 5: (GFR <15 mL/min) End Stage CKD.

1.7 How to identify kidney disease?

Your doctor will begin by inquiring about your family's medical history, the medications you're currently taking, and whether you're urinating more or less frequently than usual. Then, a physical examination will be performed.

You might also have:

- blood tests to determine the level of waste products in your system
- urine test to detect renal failure
- An ultrasound is one imaging examination that enables the doctor to see your kidneys.
- A kidney biopsy involves sending kidney tissue to a lab for analysis to identify the source of your kidney problems.

1.8 Can Kidney Disease Be Cured?

Doctors strive to help you regulate your cholesterol, blood sugar, and blood pressure levels as part of the treatment for kidney disease, which places more emphasis on addressing the disease's underlying causes. These techniques can also be used to treat kidney disease.

- ○ **Medication and Drugs**

Angiotensin receptor blockers (ARBs), such as irbesartan and olmesartan, and angiotensin-converting enzymes (ACE) inhibitors, such as ramipril and lisinopril, or cholesterol medications, such as simvastatin, are some of the prescription types that your doctor may give. These drugs aid in reducing the progression of renal disease. Your physician may still recommend these drugs even if you don't have increased blood pressure to maintain renal function.

- ○ **Changes to Your Diet And Lifestyle**

By adopting a healthy lifestyle, you can reduce your risk of developing kidney disease or any of its underlying causes. As vital as taking medication is, adopting a healthy lifestyle is.

Your physician might advise you to:

- Start eating entire grains, fresh fruit, low-fat dairy, and vegetables to promote heart health.
- Reduce weight.
- Boost your physical activity
- Give up smoking and consume less booze
- Reduce your salt intake.
- Eat fewer foods that are high in cholesterol.
- Diabetes can be managed with insulin injections

1.9 <u>Can renal illness be prevented?</u>

The first step in preventing kidney disease is to schedule routine visits with your doctor throughout your life. In the US, renal illness poses a risk to about one in three persons. Determine and address any kidney disease risk factors.

- ○ Organize your hypertension. Their blood pressure should

be 120/80.

- If you have diabetes, control your blood sugar levels.
- Adopt a balanced diet. Consume a diet low in salt and fat.
- Avoid smoking.
- Be active for at least 30 minutes 5 days a week.
- Keep a healthy weight.
- Only use over-the-counter painkillers as indicated. Your kidneys could be harmed if you take more than is recommended.

Chapter 2: The Renal Diet

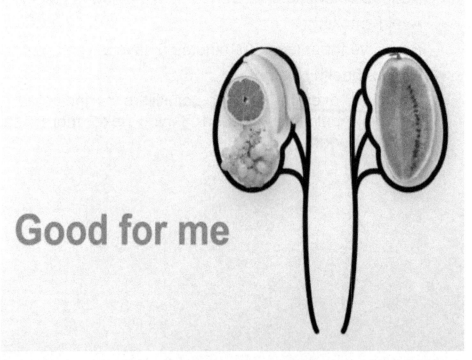

You can keep your body running on the fuel it needs by taking in the right kinds of food and liquids. The kidneys get anything the body does not require through the blood.

The kidneys produce urine and filter out extra nutrients. Some nutrients can accumulate and harm your kidneys if you have renal disease. You can prevent kidney damage with a renal diet.

2.1 Renal diet: what is it?

For people with kidney disease, a renal diet helps maintain good kidney function. Under your ribs, on each side of your spine, are the bean-shaped kidneys. They carry out crucial tasks like:

- Filtration of blood.
- Using urine to remove waste.

- Preserving the balance of fluids in your body.

Your kidneys are unable to filter your blood as they normally would if you have kidney disease. This enables an excessive buildup of salt, phosphorus, potassium, and protein waste products in your blood. This could exacerbate renal impairment and lead to excessive fluid retention in your body.

Protein, salt, potassium, and phosphorus are all reduced on a renal diet. Your kidneys are protected, which means they won't have to work as hard. Additionally, it helps with fluid control to prevent fluid retention.

Depending on how severe your kidney disease is, your recommended daily intake of phosphorus, protein, salt, and potassium will vary. Your doctor will advise you on when and how much to restrict if you suffer from advanced renal disease.

2.2 **Foods to include in a renal diet**

Fresh and whole foods are preferable to frozen, packaged, or canned foods when following a renal diet. Because whole meals have a more concentrated amount of nutrients and contain less salt by nature, whole foods are superior for the health of your kidneys as well as the rest of your body.

Meals with a range of low-potassium fruits, lean protein foods and veggies, and whole grains are simple to make with a little planning.

Protein choices

While getting sufficient protein is crucial for keeping healthy kidneys, too much protein can be harmful when your kidneys aren't functioning properly. A little portion of protein is typically acceptable at every meal. You can ask a dietitian for advice on how much to eat.

Several good sources of protein are:

- turkey or Chicken (without skin))

- Fish or seafood.
- Lean beef, such as tenderloin or sirloin.
- Eggs.
- Beans such as lentils or kidney beans and tofu. Keep in mind that because they have more phosphorus and potassium, you might want to restrict the amount you eat.

Vegetable and fruit options

Due to their high potassium content, fruits and vegetables may have to be avoided or eaten in moderation. Working with a renal dietician is recommended since they can advise you on what and how much to consume. There are several delicious fruits and veggies with lower potassium content, including:

- Blueberries
- Apples
- Blackberries
- Cabbage
- Cherries
- Green beans
- Grapes
- Pineapple
- Sweet peppers
- Strawberries
- Tangerines
- Kale
- Cucumbers
- Eggplant
- Lettuce
- Zucchini

Choices for starches and grains

Most whole grains contain potassium, but they also contain fiber, vitamins, and minerals. You may have to reduce your intake of whole grains and portion sizes. Some wholesome options with less potassium include:

- Buckwheat
- Bulgur
- Barley
- Wild rice
- Unsalted popcorn
- The potassium content of white bread, pasta, and rice is lower than that of whole-grain products. If these are preferable choices for you, ask your dietitian.

2.3 <u>Foods to omit from a renal diet</u>

Most convenience foods, whether packaged or canned, are quite rich in salt. The same is true of pickled vegetables and processed or seasoned meats. Choose items with less sodium than 240 mg per serving by reading the nutrition information label.

You should restrict or avoid consuming these sodium-rich foods:

- Crackers, pretzels, popcorn, and chips.
- Soups or stews in cans.
- Olives, pickled vegetables, and pickled relishes.
- Hot dogs, bacon, and sausages from the deli, unless they specifically state that they are "low sodium."
- Packaged meals, such as mac and cheese or frozen entrees.
- Prepared rice or noodles in a package.
- Frozen seasoned fish or meats, such as fish sticks or chicken strips.

Limit these items high in potassium as well:

- Apricots.
- Bananas.
- Dried fruits
- Honeydew.
- Spinach.
- Cantaloupe.
- Kiwi.
- Oranges.
- Carrots.
- Parsnips.
- Broccoli.
- Potatoes (sweet and white).
- Winter squash.
- Tomatoes (and tomato juice or sauce).
- Nuts and nut butter.
- Seeds like pumpkin or sunflower seeds.
- Molasses.
- Chocolate.
- Bran cereal and granola.
- Potassium-rich alternatives to salt.

On a renal diet, you might have to limit your intake of these high-phosphorus foods:

- Dairy products include ice cream, milk, yogurt, and cheese.
- Dried beans like pinto, kidney, or black beans.
- Mushrooms.

- Cocoa.
- Beer.
- Dark soft drinks, such as root beers or colas.

Milk and oat milk alternatives are getting more and more popular. The amount of phosphorus in oat milk varies by brand and can reach 20%.

You can learn from a nutritionist how many milligrams of salt, potassium, and phosphorus is in your diet. You can eat these meals regularly, or you can eat them rarely and in little amounts, depending on how healthy your kidneys are.

2.4 <u>Why is it beneficial to follow the renal diet?</u>

Patients with failing kidneys—typically because of kidney disease—are often prescribed a kidney diet. For individuals who require dialysis, doctors frequently suggest a kidney diet.

An improved sense of wellness for the patient, reduced strain on the kidneys, and relief from kidney disease symptoms are all advantages of a kidney diet, often called a kidney diet. Additionally, the diet seeks to delay kidney failure in patients.

Since the kidneys perform a crucial job, it is crucial to keep them in good condition or to operate at their best.

People may believe that the kidneys' only function is to aid in the removal of urine and some other waste products from the body, such as toxins and ammonia, but they also play a role in the production of RBC (red blood cells) and maintaining stable blood pressure. These organs use around one-fifth of the blood flow in the body to perform all this job.

Since there are risks involved, doctors' guidance is strongly recommended before starting this kind of diet for persons with kidney issues. However, the medical community frequently believes that the advantages outweigh the hazards.

If such a diet is advised by a doctor, failing to adhere to it could cause renal failure to proceed or develop. To better understand their bodies' needs and create an eating strategy they can stick to, patients are frequently encouraged to speak with a specialized nutritionist known as a renal dietitian. A renal dietician can also point patients in the direction of the right vitamins for their bodies.

For persons with renal issues, the amounts of protein, potassium, and phosphorus in the body are particularly important. The balance of these compounds can get off if the kidneys aren't functioning properly, which can lead to significant sickness.

By making sure there isn't too much phosphorus present, the renal diet aids a patient in maintaining bone strength while limiting protein to the right quantity. A patient's heartbeat may be adversely impacted by too much potassium.

A kidney diet can assist control the body's salt level, which is also of particular significance for someone with kidney issues. If patients don't pay attention to their salt intake and the volume of liquid they consume, they won't be able to eliminate enough fluid from their bodies.

Inadequate sodium and fluid consumption can lead to fluid retention and swelling, which can cause pain in places like the legs if they aren't treated. This is particularly true when kidney disease is advanced.

2.5 <u>Cooking tips for renal diets</u>

It's important to check food labels and ingredient lists, as well as renal diet shopping lists, to find any things you should stay away from. For ideas on nutritious meals and snacks, you might wish to invest in cookbooks that are good for your kidneys. Inquire about resources and suggestions from your nutritionist.

Try the following cooking advice to lower the salt and potassium content of your meals:

When flavoring or preparing food, avoid using salt or salt substitutes containing potassium chloride. Instead, use salt-free herb blends, fresh, dried, or dried herbs to flavor your cuisine. Other excellent taste enhancers are citrus zest, onions, garlic, mustard, and flavored vinegar.

Choose reduced sodium or versions with no added salt when purchasing canned goods like beans, veggies, or tuna. To further decrease salt, drain and wash the vegetables in a colander.

Foods high in potassium, such as potatoes and winter squash, can be lowered in your daily intake by chopping them up and soaking them in a lot of water. When you're ready to cook, pour out the water and put in new water. Then bring the pot to a boil.

Instead of fresh fruit, use canned fruits that have been packed in water. Before consuming the fruit, make sure to drain out the water.

It takes some getting used to shopping and preparing meals for a renal diet. However, once you master it, it will come naturally. You'll be able to prepare meals that are both nutritious and delectable with practice and support.

2.6 <u>Most common questions</u>

○ **Do protein-rich diets lead to kidney disease?**

People with early kidney disease may have worse kidney function if they eat a lot of protein. A protein diet is not hazardous for most people with healthy kidneys, especially if it is followed for a brief length of time. The long-term effects of eating a diet strong in protein and low in carbohydrates are still being researched.

○ **Does soda damage my kidneys?**

Except for most root beer brands, many dark drinks should be avoided. They have ingredients that are 100 percent absorbed by the body, including phosphorus. Make sure to look for phosphorus-containing substances on food labels.

Dark drinks can be swapped out for acceptable root beers, 7UP, cream soda, Cherry 7UP, ginger ale, and Sprite. Even though these drinks have lower phosphorus content, it is still advisable to restrict your soda consumption to avoid consuming too many empty calories, as soda has no nutritional benefit.

- **What types of vegetables may I consume if I have stage 3 chronic renal disease?**

You have little kidney damage if your chronic kidney disease is stage 3. If blood tests reveal that you have elevated potassium levels, it's crucial to limit certain veggies. Broccoli, asparagus, celery, cauliflower, cucumbers, eggplant, and fresh spinach are a few of the greatest veggies to eat. Make careful to limit portions to 1/2 cup with two to three daily servings.

- **Is it acceptable to occasionally eat low-sodium cold cuts or hot dogs for lunch?**

Portion sizes are crucial in regulating your phosphorus consumption because foods like deli meats and hot dogs are high in phosphorus. For instance, including deli meats and hot dogs a few times per month may be okay for you if your phosphorus content is constantly below or below aim.

- **Can people with renal problems eat certain types of cheese?**

Phosphorus is found in considerable quantities in cheese. Cream cheese, Swiss, natural cheddar, and Brie are among the cheeses that have lower phosphorus content than others. The typical recommendation for cheese consumption on a low-phosphorus diet is one to two ounces.

- **What kind of eating regimen should I follow following a kidney transplant?**

Since every transplant is unique, your doctor and a renal dietitian will be able to better advise you about which foods to add to your diet as you advance, thanks to your blood work.

Protein needs are increased following a transplant because of increased wound healing and steroid drug doses required to suppress the immune system. If you have diabetes, steroid drugs may cause your blood sugar to rise.

You can regulate your blood sugar with assistance from your physician or a diabetes educator. Your need for calcium will rise due to the larger dose of steroid drugs. Therefore you should concentrate on eating foods high in calcium to maintain healthy bones. In general, unless otherwise advised by your medical staff, you should keep eating a low-sodium diet.

To make sure you're getting enough minerals like phosphorus and magnesium, it's frequently advised to eat more bran, whole grains, beans, nuts & seeds, and lentils. Finally, it's critical to minimize unintended weight gain after transplant because of greater desire, improved food palatability, and fewer dietary limitations. If you're interested in dietary guidance for the best health, ask your doctor to recommend a renal dietitian.

Chapter 3: Breakfast recipes for a renal diet

A healthy breakfast sets you up for a productive morning. Breakfast may be a wonderful way to include wholesome and delectable items and get your day off to a good start. What about a nutritious renal diet breakfast, though? Let's examine the components of a nutritious renal diet breakfast, various breakfast suggestions, and packaged foods that can be included.

3.1 Scrambled eggs with cheese and fresh herbs

- ◦ Preparation time: 15 minutes
- ◦ Cooking time: 10 minutes
- ◦ Serving: 4

Ingredients

- ◦ Egg whites
- ◦ Eggs
- ◦ ¼ cup of unsweetened rice milk
- ◦ ½ cup of cream cheese
- ◦ 1 tablespoon of tarragon, chopped fresh
- ◦ 1 tablespoon of scallion, finely chopped, only the green part
- ◦ 2 tablespoons of butter, unsalted
- ◦ Freshly ground black pepper

Directions:

- ◦ Eggs, cream cheese, egg whites, scallions, rice milk, and tarragon should all be thoroughly combined and smooth in a medium bowl.

- Melt the butter in a wide skillet over moderate heat, swirling to evenly coat the pan.
- Add the egg mixture, constantly stirring for about 5 minutes or until the curds are creamy and the eggs are thick. Sprinkle with pepper.

Nutritional facts: Calories 221; Fat: 19g; Carbs: 3g; Protein: 8g; Sodium: 193mg; Potassium: 140mg; Phosphorus: 119mg

<u>3.2</u> <u>Loaded Vegetable Eggs</u>

- Preparation time: 5 minutes
- Cooking time: 10 minutes
- Serving: 2

Ingredients

- 4 whole eggs
- 1 cup of fresh spinach
- 1 cup of cauliflower
- 1 minced garlic clove
- ¼ cup of chopped onion
- 1 tablespoon of coconut/avocado oil
- ¼ teaspoon of black pepper
- ¼ cup bell pepper, chopped
- A spring onion and fresh parsley for garnish

Directions:

- Eggs and pepper should be beaten until light and fluffy.
- In a large skillet, heat the oil over medium heat.
- Cook the peppers in the skillet with the onions until they are transparent and golden.
- Add garlic, stir quickly to mix, and then add cauliflower and

spinach right away.

- Sauté the vegetables, then reduce the heat to moderate and cover for five minutes.
- Add the eggs and mix them into the veggies.
- Add some spring onions or chopped parsley on top once the eggs are done cooking. If there is not any potassium restriction, feel free to present with a side of fresh, vibrant tomatoes sprinkled with coarse black pepper. It would also be nice to add some feta or a strong, sharp cheese to them.

Nutritional facts: Calories 240; Fat: 17g; Carbs: 9g; Protein: 15g; Sodium: 194mg; Potassium: 616mg; Phosphorus: 108mg

<u>3.3</u>   <u>Chai apple smoothie</u>

- Preparation time: 5 minutes
- Cooking time: 5 minutes
- Serving: 2

Ingredients

- 1 cup of unsweetened rice milk
- 1 chopped apple
- 1 tea bag of chai
- 1 cup of ice

Directions:

- Rice milk should be heated in a medium size saucepan over low flame for about 5 minutes or until steaming.
- Take the milk off the heat and put the tea bag in it so it can steep.
- Let the milk and tea bag cool in the fridge for about 30 minutes. Then, remove the tea bag and gently squeeze it

to get all the flavor out.

- ○ Blend the apple, ice, and milk in a blender until well combined.
- ○ Dispense into 2 glasses.

Nutritional facts: Calories 88; Fat: 1g; Carbs: 19; Protein: 1g; Sodium: 47mg; Potassium: 92mg; Phosphorus: 74mg

3.4 Berry parfait

- ○ Preparation time: 15 minutes
- ○ Cooking time: 0 minutes
- ○ Serving: 4

Ingredients

- ○ 1 cup of vanilla-rice milk
- ○ cups of blueberries
- ○ ½ cup of cream cheese
- ○ ½ teaspoon of ground cinnamon
- ○ 1 tablespoon of granulated sugar
- ○ 1 cup of crumbled Meringue Cookies
- ○ 1 cup of fresh sliced strawberries

Directions:

- ○ Whisk the milk, sugar, cream cheese, and cinnamon together until combined in a small bowl.
- ○ Spoon 1/4 cup of cookie crumbs into the bottom of 4 (6-ounce) glasses.
- ○ Spread the 1/4 cup cream cheese over the cookies.
- ○ Add 1/4 cup of berries on top of the cream cheese.
- ○ Then add the cream cheese mixture, berries, and cookies to each cup in turn.

- Serve after an hour of refrigeration.

Nutritional facts: Calories 243; Fat: 11g; Carbs: 33g; Protein: 4g; Sodium: 145mg; Potassium: 189mg; Phosphorus: 84mg

3.5   <u>Breakfast green soup</u>

- Preparation time: 5 minutes
- Cooking time: 5 minutes
- Serving: 2

Ingredients

- cups chicken or vegetable broth, low sodium
- 1 halved avocado
- 1 cup of spinach
- 1 teaspoon of ground coriander
- 1 teaspoon of ground turmeric
- 1 teaspoon of ground cumin
- Freshly ground black pepper

Directions:

- Add the avocado, spinach, broth, cumin, coriander, and turmeric to a blender until smooth, process.
- Place the mixture in a small saucepan and heat for 2 to 3 minutes or until thoroughly cooked. Sprinkle with pepper.

Nutritional facts: Calories 221; Fat: 18g; Carbs: 15g; Protein: 5g; Sodium: 170mg; Potassium: 551mg; Phosphorus: 58mg

3.6   <u>Apple-mint French toast</u>

- Preparation time: 2 minutes
- Cooking time: 5 minutes
- Serving: 2

Ingredients

- Lightly beaten eggs
- ¾ cup (175 ml) of applesauce
- 1/8 teaspoon (1/2 ml) of mint
- ½ cup (125 ml) of milk
- white bread, slices

Directions:

- In a bowl, whisk together the milk, eggs, and mint. Add the apple sauce.
- Melt some olive oil in a nonstick pan over medium-high heat.
- Take a piece of bread, dip it in the mixture, and repeat with the remaining slices.
- The bottom of moistened bread slices should be browned in the pan before flipping to fry the other side.
- Serve with syrup on top.

Nutritional facts: Calories 352; Fat: 17g; Carbs: 60g; Protein: 12g; Sodium: 462mg; Potassium: 254mg; Phosphorus: 184mg

<u>3.7</u> <u>Hot multigrain cereal</u>

- Preparation time: 5 minutes
- Cooking time: 30 minutes
- Serving: 1

Ingredients

- 3/4 cup of water
- 1 tablespoon (steel-cut) oats, uncooked
- 1 tablespoon of old-fashioned and uncooked grits
- 1 tablespoon of uncooked (roasted) whole buckwheat

- ◦ 1 tablespoon of uncooked bulgur
- ◦ 1 tablespoon of uncooked couscous

Directions:

- ◦ In a covered 1-1/2-quart pot, boil water.
- ◦ Grits should be added, then quickly stirred.
- ◦ Shortly stir in the bulgur, buckwheat, and oats.
- ◦ Reduce flame to a vigorous simmer and thoroughly coat the simmering surface with nonstick cooking spray.
- ◦ Cook for 25 minutes with the lid on.
- ◦ Take the pot off the heat and add the couscous.
- ◦ After 8 minutes of covered rest, serve the pot.

Nutritional facts: Calories 150; Fat: 1g; Carbs: 30g; Protein: 5g; Sodium: 135mg; Potassium: 224mg; Phosphorus: 104mg

3.8   <u>Morning herb rolls</u>

- ◦ Preparation time: 10 minutes
- ◦ Cooking time: 25 minutes
- ◦ Serving: 18

Ingredients

- ◦ ½ cup of milk
- ◦ 1 large egg, beaten
- ◦ 1 tablespoon of sugar
- ◦ 1 tablespoon of canola oil
- ◦ 1 package of dry yeast
- ◦ ½ cups of flour
- ◦ 1 tablespoon of herb mix (chives, thyme, rosemary, and parsley)

Directions:

- Allow yeast to settle for 5 minutes in 1/4 cup of tepid water.
- Put the sugar into the water in the cup.
- Mix the flour, milk, herbs, canola oil, and milk in a bowl.
- Beat the egg and add it to the dough. Save 1 tsp of the beaten egg for later.
- Mix dough thoroughly.
- On a flat surface, sprinkle flour and knead the dough until it is elastic for about 10 minutes.
- Form kneaded dough into balls that are (1/2 oz) about 1 1/2 inch crosswise.
- Transfer dough balls to a refrigerator to chill overnight if desired.
- Transfer the dough rolls to a cookie sheet that has been oiled, and then wait for them to double in size for about an hour.
- The oven should be heated to 350°F.
- The rolls should be covered with the reserved beaten egg and baked for 20 to 25 minutes or until golden brown.

Nutritional facts: Calories 117; Fat: 10g; Carbs: 21; Protein: 3g; Sodium: 8mg; Potassium: 75mg; Phosphorus: 43mg

<u>3.9</u> <u>Buckwheat pancakes</u>

- Preparation time: 10 minutes
- Cooking time: 15 minutes
- Serving: 4

Ingredients

- 1 large-size egg
- 1¾ cups of unsweetened rice milk

- 1 cup of buckwheat flour
- 1 teaspoon of white vinegar
- 1½ tablespoon of sugar
- ½ cup all-purpose flour
- 1 teaspoon of vanilla extract
- 1 teaspoon of baking powder
- 2 tablespoons of butter, divided

Directions:

- Combine the vinegar and rice milk in a small bowl. Sit for five minutes.
- In the meantime, combine the all-purpose flour and buckwheat flour in a large basin. Stir in the baking powder and sugar to combine.
- Mix the rice milk with the vanilla and egg after adding them. Stir to combine the dry ingredients with the wet components.
- Melt 1 ½ teaspoons of butter in a large pan over medium heat. The batter should be poured into the skillet using a 14-cup measuring cup. Cook the pancakes for 2 - 3 minutes or until they start to bubble slightly. Cook for one to two minutes on the other side before flipping.
- Place the cooked pancakes on a serving dish and continue cooking the batter in the skillet in batches, using more butter as necessary.

Nutritional facts: Calories 281; Fat: 9g; Carbs: 43g; Protein: 7g; Sodium: 232mg; Potassium: 339mg; Phosphorus: 147mg

3.10 Leek and Brussels sprout quiche

- Preparation time: 20 minutes
- Cooking time: 1 hour

- Serving: 4

Ingredients
For crust:
- ¾ cup (unbleached) flour
- 5 tablespoons (unsalted) butter, frozen and cubed
- 1 pinch of sea salt
- 2-3 tablespoons of ice water

For filling:
- Medium eggs
- 1 tablespoons unsalted butter
- 170g Brussels sprouts, thinly slice
- 120g leek, thinly sliced
- 2 tablespoons of tarragon leaves, chopped
- ounces of goat cheese
- ¾ cup of whole milk
- ⅓ cup of heavy cream
- ¼ teaspoon of freshly ground black pepper

Directions:
- To make the crust, heat the oven to 350°F.
- In a medium bowl, mix the flour and salt.
- Using a fork, pastry cutter, or your fingertips, cut 5 tbsp of butter in the flour mixture until the mixture forms coarse pea-sized pieces.
- Add one tablespoon of cold water at a time. Make a cohesive dough by combining it with your hands.
- Take the dough and place it on a floured surface. Knead

the dough until the ball forms.

- With the use of a rolling pin, form the dough into a 12-inch round, 14-inch thick circle.
- Place the rolled-out dough on a 9-inch pie plate by gently pressing it down.
- With your fingers, crimp the crust's edges. Use a fork to prick the dough's bottom.
- The dough in the pan should be covered with parchment paper. To make the dough more compact, lay baking weights or dried beans on parchment paper.
- Bake the pastry for around 20 minutes or until it is halfway done. Take out of the oven, then let cool for ten minutes.
- Melt tbsp of butter in a big skillet over medium heat for the filling and assembling. Add tarragon, leeks, and Brussels sprouts.
- Reduce the flame and cook the brussels sprouts and leeks for around 10 minutes or until they are almost cooked through. Place aside.
- In a big mixing bowl, combine the eggs, milk, and cream and whisk to combine.
- Add goat cheese crumbles to the mixture. Use pepper to season.
- Fill the pie crust with the Brussels sprout and leek mixture evenly.
- Pour the mixture of eggs and cheese on top.
- To get a set custard, bake for roughly 40 minutes.

Nutritional facts: Calories 260; Fat: 19g; Carbs: 15g; Protein: 8g; Sodium: 232mg; Potassium: 339mg; Phosphorus: 147mg

<u>3.11</u>　　　　　<u>Chia pudding</u>

- Preparation time: 10 minutes
- Cooking time: 0 minutes
- Serving: 4

Ingredients

- ½ cup chia seeds
- ¼ teaspoon cinnamon
- 1 teaspoon vanilla extract
- 1 ½ cups of rice milk
- ¼ cup maple syrup

Directions:

- Combine the rice milk, vanilla, chia seeds, maple syrup, and cinnamon in a mason jar or bowl.
- Chia seeds should not stick to the container's sides when you stir the mixture of chia seeds until it is thoroughly combined. For at least four hours or overnight, cover and place in the refrigerator.
- Before serving, you can include fruit.

Nutritional facts: Calories 206; Fat: 4g; Carbs: 32g; Protein: 7g; Sodium: 34mg; Potassium: 236mg; Phosphorus: 85mg

3.12 Mexican breakfast eggs on toast

- Preparation time: 5 minutes
- Cooking time: 15 minutes
- Serving: 8

Ingredients

- 8 eggs, beaten
- ½ cup onion, chopped

- ○ cloves garlic, crushed
- ○ 1 ½ cups corn, frozen and thawed
- ○ 1 tablespoon of margarine
- ○ 1 ½ teaspoon ground cumin
- ○ 1/8 teaspoon of cayenne pepper
- ○ 8 toasted bread slices

Directions:

- ○ In a large skillet, melt the margarine and cook the garlic and onions until the onion is soft.
- ○ Add the cayenne, cumin, and corn. Stir it.
- ○ Add the eggs and cook them over low heat, occasionally stirring, until they are set.
- ○ Place the toasted bread slices on the dish, then top with the egg mixture.

Nutritional facts: Calories 214; Fat: 8g; Carbs: 13g; Protein: 9g; Sodium: 234mg; Potassium: 107mg; Phosphorus: 100mg

3.13 Stuffed omelet with vegetables

- ○ Preparation time: 10 minutes
- ○ Cooking time: 8 minutes
- ○ Serving: 1

Ingredients

- ○ 1 ounce of cheddar cheese (low fat), shredded sharp
- ○ 1 (large) egg whites
- ○ 1 large egg, whole
- ○ 2 tablespoons water
- ○ 1/3 cup zucchini, chopped

- tablespoons green onions, chopped
- ¼ teaspoon of black pepper
- ¼ cup (whole-kernel) corn, frozen and thawed

Directions:

- A frying pan should be heated at high-medium heat. Spray cooking oil on the pan.
- Add zucchini, onions, and corn, and cook the vegetables for 4 minutes or until they are crisp-tender. Turn off the heat.
- A 10-inch nonstick skillet should be heated over high to medium heat.
- Egg, water, egg whites, and pepper are combined in a bowl and thoroughly whisked.
- Cook the egg mixture in the pan for about 2 minutes, or until the edges begin to set, after spraying the pan with cooking spray. With a spatula, gently lift the pan's sides and turn it so that the uncooked side flows to the hot surface.
- Add the vegetables to the bottom half of the omelet before topping it with strong cheddar cheese.
- To fold an omelet in half, loosen the sides with a spatula. The cheese needs an additional two minutes of cooking. Place on a dish, then savor.

Nutritional facts: Calories 187; Fat: 12g; Carbs: 11g; Protein: 22g; Sodium: 270mg; Potassium: 352mg; Phosphorus: 218mg

3.14   Breakfast burrito with green chilies

- Preparation time: 10 minutes
- Cooking time: 8 minutes
- Serving: 2

Ingredients

- 4 eggs
- ½ teaspoon hot pepper sauce
- 2 tablespoons salsa
- 1 tablespoons of diced green chilies
- ¼ teaspoon of ground cumin
- 2 flour tortillas

Directions:

- Over medium heat, coat a medium-sized skillet with nonstick cooking spray.
- In a bowl, combine green chilies, eggs, spicy sauce, and cumin.
- Once the skillet is heated, pour the egg mixture in, and cook while stirring for one to two minutes or until the egg is set.
- Toasted tortillas should be heated in another pan or microwave for 20 seconds.
- Each tortilla should have 1/2 an egg on it before being rolled up burrito-style.
- Serve with a tablespoon of salsa.

Nutritional facts: Calories 225; Fat: 16g; Carbs: 1.3g; Protein: 13g; Sodium: 296mg; Potassium: 195mg; Phosphorus: 122mg

3.15 <u>Blueberry pancakes</u>

- Preparation time: 5 minutes
- Cooking time: 5 minutes
- Serving: 6

Ingredients

- 1 egg, slightly beaten
- 1 cup blueberries, canned/frozen and rinsed
- 1 cup buttermilk
- 2 teaspoons baking powder
- 2 tablespoons sugar
- 2 tablespoons (no-salt) margarine, melted
- 1 ½ cups all-purpose flour, sifted

Directions:

- In a mixing basin, sift together the flour, sugar, and baking powder.
- Create a hole in the center and add the remaining ingredients.
- To create a smooth batter, begin stirring in the middle and add the dry ingredients slowly.
- A 12-inch heavy skillet or griddle should be lightly greased. Spoon 1/3 cup of the batter into the heated skillet, cook until the underside is browned, then flip it over and toast the other side.

Nutritional facts: Calories 223; Fat: 20g; Carbs: 33g; Protein: 7g; Sodium: 196mg; Potassium: 128mg; Phosphorus: 100mg

3.16   Egg and avocado bake

- Preparation time: 5 minutes
- Cooking time: 15 minutes
- Serving: 2

Ingredients

- 2 large eggs
- 1 avocado, halved

- 1 tablespoon parsley, chopped
- Freshly ground black pepper

Directions:
- The oven should be preheated at 425 °F .
- Carefully crack one egg into a small basin while preserving the yolk.
- The avocado halves should be placed cut-side up on a baking pan. Fill one half with the egg. Repeat with the remaining avocado and egg halves. Use pepper to season.
- Bake the egg for 15 minutes or until it is set. After removing from the oven, top with fresh parsley. Serve.

Nutritional facts: Calories 242; Fat: 20g; Carbs: 9g; Protein: 9g; Sodium: 88mg; Potassium: 575mg; Phosphorus: 164mg

<u>3.17 Broccoli-basil quiche</u>

- Preparation time: 10 minutes
- Cooking time: 55 minutes
- Serving: 8

Ingredients
- 1 egg, beaten
- 1 frozen pie crust, store-bought
- 1 tomato, chopped
- 2 scallions, chopped
- 2 cups broccoli, finely chopped
- 2 tablespoons basil, chopped
- ½ cup feta cheese, crumbled
- 1 tablespoon of all-purpose flour

- ○ 1 clove garlic, minced
- ○ 1 cup of rice milk
- ○ Freshly ground black pepper

Directions:

- ○ The oven should be preheated at 425°F.
- ○ The pie crust should be used to line a pie pan. Fork-prick the crust numerous times. The crust should bake for 10 minutes. Take the food out of the oven and lower the heat to 325°F.
- ○ Broccoli, scallions, tomato, feta, garlic, eggs, rice milk, basil, and flour should all be combined in a medium bowl. Use pepper to season.
- ○ In the pie pan that has been made, pour the broccoli and egg mixture. Until a knife placed in the center of the cake comes out clean, bake for 35 - 45 minutes. Before serving, allow it to cool for 10 - 15 minutes.

Nutritional facts: Calories 160; Fat: 10g; Carbs: 13g; Protein: 6g; Sodium: 252mg; Potassium: 175mg; Phosphorus: 101mg

3.18   Asparagus frittata

- ○ Preparation time: 5 minutes
- ○ Cooking time: 30 minutes
- ○ Serving: 2

Ingredients

- ○ 4 large eggs
- ○ 1 teaspoon of (extra-virgin) olive oil divided
- ○ 10 (medium) asparagus spears, ends trimmed
- ○ Freshly ground black pepper

- ¼ cup parsley, chopped
- ½ teaspoon of onion powder

Directions:
- Set the oven's temperature to 450 degrees Fahrenheit.
- Add pepper and 1 tsp of olive oil to the asparagus before tossing.
- Transfer it to a baking tray, and roast for 20 minutes, tossing periodically or till the spears are soft and browned.
- Beat the eggs together with the parsley and onion powder in a small bowl.
- Use pepper to season.
- Arrange the asparagus spears inside a medium skillet after cutting each spear into 1-inch sections. Shake the pan to spread the remaining oil before adding it.
- Place the skillet over medium heat and add the egg mixture. When the egg is nearly set on top but completely set on the bottom, cover it with the plate, flip the frittata over onto the plate, then put it again in the pan with the fried side facing up. Cook for a further 30 to 60 seconds or until firm.

Nutritional facts: Calories 102; Fat: 8g; Carbs: 4g; Protein: 6g; Sodium: 46mg; Potassium: 248mg; Phosphorus: 103mg

3.19 Corn pudding

- Preparation time: 10 minutes
- Cooking time: 40 minutes
- Serving: 6

Ingredients
- 3 eggs

- Unsalted butter for greasing
- ½ teaspoon baking soda
- 2 tablespoons of all-purpose flour
- ¾ cup rice milk, unsweetened
- 3 tablespoons (unsalted) butter, melted
- 2 tablespoons sugar, granulated
- 2 tablespoons cream, light sour

Directions:

- Set the oven's temperature to 350 °F.
- Butter an 8-by-8-inch baking dish then set it aside.
- Flour and the baking soda substitute should be combined in a small basin and left aside.
- Whisk the eggs, butter, rice milk, sour cream, and sugar in a medium bowl.
- The flour mixture should be smoothly incorporated into the egg mixture.
- Stir the corn into the batter until it is thoroughly combined.
- Bake for around 40 minutes, or till the pudding is set, after ladling the mixture into the baking dish.
- Serve the pudding warm after it has cooled for about 15 minutes.

Nutritional facts: Calories 175; Fat: 10g; Carbs: 19g; Protein: 5g; Sodium: 62mg; Potassium: 170mg; Phosphorus: 101mg

3.20 Breakfast wrap with fruit and cheese

- Preparation time: 10 minutes
- Cooking time: 0 minutes
- Serving: 2

Ingredients

- 2 tablespoons cream cheese
- 2 (6-inch) flour tortillas
- 1 tablespoon of honey
- 1 apple, sliced thin

Directions:

- Spread 1 tbsp of cream cheese over each tortilla, leaving approximately 1/2 inch around the borders, and place both tortillas on a spotless work area.
- On the tortilla's side that is closest to you, place the apple slices upon the cream cheese, leaving approximately 11/2 inches on either side and 2" on the bottom.
- Lightly drizzle some honey over the apples.
- Laying the edge of the tortilla over the apples, fold the right and left edges toward the center.
- Fold the edge of the tortilla closest to you over the side pieces and the fruit. The tortilla should be rolled away from you to form a tight wrap.
- The second tortilla should then be used.

Nutritional facts: Calories 188; Fat: 6g; Carbs: 33g; Protein: 4g; Sodium: 177mg; Potassium: 136mg; Phosphorus: 73mg

Chapter 4:   Salads and Soups

Salads and soups are classic pairings that are suitable for any season. When on a renal diet, there are lots of meaty and lighter options to enjoy. Soups and salads are a great way to creatively include vegetables and fruits in your diet, in addition to increasing your protein consumption and providing fiber.

4.1 Beef barley soup with vegetables

- ◊ Preparation time: 5 minutes
- ◊ Cooking time: 1 hour 30 minutes
- ◊ Serving: 7

Ingredients

- ◊ ½ teaspoon black pepper
- ◊ ¼ cup vegetable oil
- ◊ ½ cup mushrooms, sliced
- ◊ 1 cup onion, chopped
- ◊ 2 carrots, diced
- ◊ 3 cups water
- ◊ ¼ teaspoon dried thyme
- ◊ ½ teaspoon garlic, minced
- ◊ 14.5 ounces of low sodium chicken broth
- ◊ 1 package (16 ounces) vegetables frozen
- ◊ ½ cup barley
- ◊ 2 potatoes, diced

Directions:

- ◊ Add pepper to beef.

- Add 2 TBSP oil to a stew pot and cook for 5 minutes.
- Add 2 additional tablespoons of oil along with the mushrooms, onions, and carrots.
- Stir frequently for about five minutes.
- Add the garlic and thyme and cook for three minutes.
- Fill the pot with water and chicken broth.
- Add barley, potatoes, and a variety of veggies.
- Stir and heat to a boil.
- Cover and turn down the heat
- Simmer for 1 1/2 to 2 hours.

Nutritional facts:
- Calories 270
- Fat: 0g
- Carbs: 22g
- Protein: 23g

4.2 Kohlrabi soup

- Preparation time: 10 minutes
- Cooking time: 35 minutes
- Serving: 12

Ingredients
- 1 pound of kohlrabies, cut into chunks
- 1 pound celeriac, cut into chunks
- 2 tablespoons butter
- 2 quarts chicken broth, low salt
- ½ pound potatoes, cut into chunks
- 1 cup onions, chopped

- 1 cup of light cream
- Ground pepper, as required
- Pinch nutmeg

Directions:
- The oven should be heated to 400°F.
- Bake potatoes in a hot oven until they are soft.
- Wait until it cools.
- Scoop out the pulp from lengthwise-cut potatoes.
- Over medium heat, add the flour and slowly whisk in the milk until thoroughly incorporated.
- Fill the flour mixture with pepper and potato pulp.
- Stir until thick and bubbling.
- Add the cheese and continue stirring until it melts.
- Turn off the heat, add the sour cream, and mix until combined.

Nutritional facts:
- Calories 180
- Fat: 4g
- Carbs: 20g
- Protein: 8g

4.3 Soup with rotisserie chicken noodles
- Preparation time: 10 minutes
- Cooking time: 25 minutes
- Serving: 2

Ingredients

- 8 cups chicken broth, low sodium
- 1 rotisserie chicken prepared
- ½ cup onion
- 1 cup of carrots
- 1 cup of celery
- 3 tablespoons parsley
- 6 ounces of noodles, uncooked

Directions:
- Chicken should be deboned and then chopped into bite-sized pieces. For the soup, measure 4 cups.
- A large stockpot with chicken broth added should be brought to a boil.
- Slice and chop carrots, celery, and onion.
- Add chicken, veggies, and noodles to a stock pot.
- The noodles must be cooked for around 15 minutes after bringing them to a boil.
- Chop parsley leaves for garnish.

Nutritional facts:
- Calories 185
- Fat: 5g
- Carbs: 14g
- Protein: 21g

4.4 Soup with a creamy vegetable mixture

- Preparation time: 10 minutes
- Cooking time: 30 minutes
- Serving: 4

Ingredients

Soup Base:

- 2 tablespoons of avocado oil
- ½ teaspoon thyme, dried
- 1 garlic clove, roughly chopped
- 1 cup of cauliflower florets, fresh/frozen and thawed
- ½ small onion, roughly chopped
- 1½ cup of zucchini, chunks
- 1 cup of coconut milk
- 1½ cups vegetable broth, low sodium

Soup:

- 2 tablespoons of avocado oil
- 1 medium carrot, diced / grated
- ½ small onion, finely diced
- 1 stalk celery, diced
- 1 cup kale, packed
- ¼ teaspoon pepper and salt, each to taste
- 1 tablespoon of nutritional yeast (optional)
- 2 cloves garlic, finely chopped
- 1 teaspoon white wine vinegar, to taste (optional)

Directions:

- Add avocado oil to a saucepan set over medium heat to create the soup base. Add the chopped garlic and onion once it has warmed up. Sauté for about 2 minutes or until gently golden. Once fragrant, add the dried thyme and simmer for an additional 2 minutes.
- Add coconut milk, vegetable broth, zucchini, and

cauliflower florets.

- When the zucchini and cauliflower are both extremely tender, reduce the heat, close the lid, and let it simmer for 12 to 15 minutes.
- Use an immersion blender to purée the soup base, or let it cool slightly and then puree it in a blender until smooth and thick. Place aside.
- Avocado oil should be warmed in a spotless pan or pot. Cook the finely diced celery, onion, and carrots for about 5 minutes or until they are tender and fragrant.
- Embrace minced garlic. Stir the food while it cooks for about a minute or until it smells good. Be careful, and the garlic should not burn.
- Then add the kale and the pureed soup base. Simmer for 5 more minutes, soft the kale, and let the flavors come together. Before serving, season to taste with salt, pepper, nutritional yeast optionally, and vinegar.

Nutritional facts:
- Calories 277
- Fat: 27g
- Carbs: 10g
- Protein: 3g

4.5   Pumpkin soup
- Preparation time: 5 minutes
- Cooking time: 30 minutes
- Serving: 7

Ingredients
- 1 garlic clove, minced

- 1 onion, minced
- 2 tablespoon brown sugar
- ¼ teaspoon salt
- 1 can (15 ounces) pumpkin puree
- 1 can (15 ounces) coconut milk, low fat
- 2 cups vegetable broth, low sodium
- ½ teaspoon coriander
- 1 teaspoon curry powder
- ½ teaspoon cinnamon, ground
- 1/8 teaspoon nutmeg, ground
- ¼ cup creamy peanut butter
- ¼ teaspoon powdered ginger
- ¼ teaspoon black pepper
- ½ cup cilantro, chopped

Directions:

- In a big saucepan, heat olive oil with onion, garlic, and brown sugar until the onion is soft.
- Add the broth, seasonings, and salt to a boil.
- The onions should be cooked for about 15 minutes, occasionally stirring, on low heat.
- Add the remaining spices, pumpkin, coconut milk, and peanut butter. Cook for 5 minutes or until heated.
- Blend the soup until it is smooth by transferring it to a blender or using an immersion blender.
- Serve with cilantro on top.

Nutritional facts:

- Calories 139

- Fat: 9g
- Carbs: 14g
- Protein: 4g

4.6   A butternut squash soup

- Preparation time: 15 minutes
- Cooking time: 25 minutes
- Serving: 5

Ingredients

- 1 cup (yellow) onion, diced
- 4 cups butternut squash, diced
- 2 cloves garlic, chopped
- ½ tablespoon olive oil
- 1 cup sweet potato, diced
- 2½ cups vegetable broth, unsalted
- 1 cup carrot, sliced
- ⅛ teaspoon nutmeg, ground

Directions:

- Over medium-high heat, cook the garlic and onions in olive oil till the onion is transparent.
- Add the remaining ingredients, bring to a boil over high heat, and then simmer for about 30 minutes, or until the carrots are easily shredded with a fork.
- Using a hand blender or a stand mixer, allow it to cool before blending.

Nutritional facts:

- Calories 121

- Fat: 2g
- Carbs: 26g
- Protein: 3g

4.7   <u>Red pepper roasted soup</u>

- Preparation time: 10 minutes
- Cooking time: 25 minutes
- Serving: 4

Ingredients

- 2 tablespoons of avocado oil
- 2 garlic cloves, minced
- 1 onion, diced
- 1 ½ cups roasted red peppers, sliced
- 2 cups vegetable broth, low sodium
- 1/3 teaspoon paprika, smoked
- 3 tablespoons homemade pesto, low sodium
- 1 cup coconut milk, canned
- ¼ teaspoon of black pepper
- Salt, to taste (optional)

Directions:

- In a pot, warm up the avocado oil over medium heat. Add the diced onion and cook for about 5 minutes or until transparent and aromatic.
- For a further minute or two, add the garlic and heat it while stirring until fragrant.
- After that, incorporate the pesto, vegetable broth, and slices of drained roasted red pepper. After bringing it to a

boil, turn down the heat and continue to simmer for 10 to 15 minutes.

- When the soup has barely begun to simmer, add the coconut milk and turn the heat off.
- Blend the soup with an immersion blender until it is smooth and creamy.
- Working in sections and being cautious not to overload the mixer with the hot mixture, you can also use a strong blender. Add the soup back into the saucepan and season with salt (only if necessary), black pepper, and smoked paprika.
- Before serving, fully reheat the soup and, at your discretion, top it with a drop of coconut milk or olive oil.

Nutritional facts:

- Calories 279
- Fat: 25g
- Carbs: 12g
- Protein: 3g

4.8 Minestrone

- Preparation time: 15 minutes
- Cooking time: 1 hour
- Serving: 6

Ingredients

- 1 cup (white) onion, diced
- 2 cups of zucchini, chopped
- 2 cups celery, chopped
- 4 cups vegetable broth, low sodium

- 3 cloves garlic, minced
- 1/2 cup wheat macaroni noodles, dry whole
- 2 tablespoons tomato paste, without or low sodium
- 1 can of garbanzo beans, drained and rinsed
- 1/2 lemon, juiced
- 2 tablespoons avocado oil
- 1 teaspoon paprika
- 1 teaspoon black pepper
- ½ teaspoon rosemary, dried

Directions:

- In a large pot, warm the avocado oil on medium heat.
- Add white onion, then cook for a while.
- Sauté carrots, celery, and garlic in a saucepan for around five minutes.
- Stir in the tomato paste, pepper, paprika, and rosemary.
- Place a lid on the pot, add the vegetable broth, and heat to a boil. When the soup reaches a boil, add the zucchini, stir it in, reduce the heat, and let it simmer for 30 to 40 minutes.
- Add lemon juice, garbanzo beans, and macaroni noodles after the vegetables are ready. Noodles need another 5–10 minutes of cooking time under cover.
- Serve and savor!

Nutritional facts:

- Calories 200
- Fat: 5g
- Carbs: 7.5g

- Protein: 6g

4.9   <u>Soup with turkey bulgur</u>

- Preparation time: 25 minutes
- Cooking time: 45 minutes
- Serving: 6

Ingredients

- ½ pound ground turkey, 93% lean, cooked
- 1 teaspoon olive oil
- ½ (sweet) onion, chopped
- 1 teaspoon garlic, minced
- ½ cup green cabbage, shredded
- 1 cup of Chicken Stock
- 4 cups water
- 1 celery stalk, chopped
- 1 carrot, sliced thin
- bay leaves, dried
- 1 teaspoon fresh sage, chopped
- ½ cup bulgur
- 2 tablespoons fresh parsley, chopped
- 1 teaspoon fresh thyme, chopped
- A Pinch of red pepper flakes
- Freshly ground black pepper

Directions:

- Over medium-high heat, pour the olive oil into a large saucepan. The turkey should be cooked through after around 5 minutes of sautéing.

- When the vegetables are tender, add the garlic and onions and sauté for around 3 minutes. Add the bulgur, water, celery, carrots, cabbage, chicken stock, and bay leaves.
- The bulgur and veggies should be soft after about 35 minutes of simmering on low heat after the soup comes to a boil.
- Add the sage, thyme, parsley, and red pepper flakes after removing the bay leaves.
- Add pepper and then serve.

Nutritional facts:
- Calories 77
- Fat: 4g
- Carbs: 2g
- Protein: 8g

4.10   Cauliflower curried soup
- Preparation time: 25 minutes
- Cooking time: 30 minutes
- Serving: 6

Ingredients
- 1 (small) sweet onion, chopped
- 1 teaspoon unsalted butter
- 1 small cauliflower head, florets
- 2 teaspoons minced garlic
- 3 cups of water or more
- ½ cup cream, light sour
- 2 teaspoons of curry powder

- 3 tablespoons fresh cilantro, chopped

Directions:
- The onion and garlic should be sautéed in the butter for approximately 3 minutes, or until softened, in a large saucepan over medium-high heat.
- Curry powder, water, and cauliflower are added.
- The soup should be brought to a boil, then simmer for 20 minutes, or till the cauliflower is soft, on low heat.
- The soup should be puréed in a food processor until it reaches the desired smoothness and creaminess (or use a big bowl and immersion blender).
- Add the cilantro and sour cream before returning the soup to the pan.
- The soup should be heated through after about 5 minutes on medium-low.

Nutritional facts:
- Calories 33
- Fat: 2g
- Carbs: 2g
- Protein: 1g

4.11 Watercress cream soup
- Preparation time: 15 minutes
- Cooking time: 1 hour 10 minutes
- Serving: 4

Ingredients
- 6 cloves garlic

- 1 teaspoon butter, unsalted
- ½ teaspoon of olive oil
- ½ (sweet) onion, chopped
- ¼ cup parsley, chopped fresh
- 4 cups watercress, chopped
- 3 cups water
- 1 tablespoon lemon juice, freshly squeezed
- ¼ cup of heavy cream
- Freshly ground black pepper

Directions:

- Set the oven's temperature to 400 °F.
- The garlic should be placed on a sheet of aluminum foil. Olive oil should be drizzled after the foil is folded into a small packet. Cook the garlic for around 20 minutes, or until it is very soft, by placing the pack in a pie pan.
- The garlic should be taken out of the oven and left to cool.
- Melt the butter in a large pot over medium-high heat. The onion should be softened after 4 minutes of sautéing. After adding, sauté the parsley and watercress for 5 minutes.
- Add the water and the roasted garlic pulp and stir. Once the soup has reached a rolling boil, turn down the heat.
- The soup should simmer for about 20 minutes or till the vegetables are tender.
- After allowing the soup to cool for around 5 minutes, add the heavy cream and purée in sections in a food processor.
- Move the soup to a pot and cook it over low flame until it is thoroughly heated.
- Add the pepper and lemon juice thereafter.

Nutritional facts:

- Calories 97
- Fat: 8g
- Carbs: 5g
- Protein: 2g

4.12 Salad with strawberries and watercress with almond dressing

- Preparation time: 15 minutes
- Cooking time: 0 minutes
- Serving: 6

Ingredients

For the dressing

- ¼ cup of olive oil
- ¼ cup of rice vinegar
- 1 tablespoon of honey
- ¼ teaspoon almond extract
- ¼ teaspoon mustard, ground
- Freshly ground black pepper

For the salad

- 2 cups green leaf lettuce, shredded
- ½ cucumber, chopped
- 2 cups watercress, roughly chopped
- ½ red onion, thinly sliced
- 1 cup strawberries, sliced

Directions:

- To make the dressing, combine the rice vinegar and olive oil in a small bowl and whisk until well combined.
- Add honey, almond flavoring, mustard, and pepper; whisk until combined.
- Making the salad: Combine the watercress, onion, green leaf lettuce, cucumber, and strawberries in a big bowl.
- Mix the salad with the dressing after pouring it over it.

Nutritional facts:
- Calories 159
- Fat: 14g
- Carbs: 9g
- Protein: 1g

4.13 Lettuce salad with asparagus and raspberries
- Preparation time: 25 minutes
- Cooking time: 0 minutes
- Serving: 4

Ingredients
- 1 cup asparagus, cut into long ribbons
- 2 cups green leaf lettuce, shredded
- 1 scallion, both (green and white) parts, sliced
- 1 tablespoon of balsamic vinegar
- 1 cup raspberries
- Freshly ground black pepper

Directions:
- Place the lettuce evenly across 4 serving plates.
- On top of the greens, place the asparagus and scallion.

- After dividing the raspberries evenly, top the salads with them.
- Salads should be dressed with balsamic vinegar.
- Add pepper to taste.

Nutritional facts:
- Calories 36
- Fat: 0g
- Carbs: 8g
- Protein: 2g

4.14   Beef ginger salad

- Preparation time: 30 minutes
- Cooking time: 10 minutes
- Serving: 6

Ingredients
For the beef
- 2 tablespoons of olive oil
- 2 tablespoons lime juice, freshly squeezed
- 1 tablespoon fresh ginger, grated
- 2 teaspoons garlic, minced
- ½ pound of flank steak

For the vinaigrette
- ¼ cup of rice vinegar
- ¼ cup of olive oil
- 1 lime zest
- 1 lime juice

- 1 tablespoon of honey
- 1 teaspoon fresh thyme, chopped

For the salad
- ½ (red) onion, thin sliced
- 4 cups green leaf lettuce, torn
- ½ cup radishes, sliced

Directions:
- Mix the olive oil, ginger, lime juice, and garlic thoroughly in a small bowl.
- Turn the flank steak in the marinade to cover both sides with the flavorful sauce.
- For an hour of marinating, wrap the bowl in plastic wrap and put it in the refrigerator.
- Take the steak out of the marinade, then throw away the marinade.
- Set a grill to medium-high heat and grill the steak, turning it once, until it is medium-done, which will take approximately 5 min per side, based on how thick the steak is.
- The steak should be taken out, placed on a cutting board, and let rest for ten min.
- Thinly slice the meat against the grain.

Nutritional facts:
- Calories 200
- Fat: 14g
- Carbs: 5g
- Protein: 8g

4.15   __Confetti farfalle salad__

- Preparation time: 30 minutes
- Cooking time: 0 minutes
- Serving: 6

Ingredients

- 2 cups farfalle pasta, cooked
- ¼ cup cucumber, finely chopped
- ¼ cup red bell pepper, finely chopped and boiled
- ¼ cup carrot, grated
- ½ scallion, finely chopped (green part only)
- 2 tablespoons (yellow bell pepper
- 1 tablespoon lemon juice, freshly squeezed
- ½ teaspoon sugar, granulated
- 1 teaspoon parsley, chopped fresh
- ½ cup Mayonnaise
- Freshly ground black pepper

Directions:

- Combine the spaghetti, cucumber, yellow pepper, red pepper, carrot, and scallion in a sizable bowl.
- Mix the lemon juice, mayonnaise, parsley, and sugar in a small bowl.
- Mix the spaghetti mixture with the dressing after adding it.
- Use pepper to season.
- Serve chilled from the refrigerator after at least one hour.

Nutritional facts:

- Calories 119

- Fat: 3g
- Carbs: 20g
- Protein: 4g

4.16 Lemon-dressed cucumber-dill salad with cabbage

- Preparation time: 25 minutes
- Cooking time: 0 minutes
- Serving: 4

Ingredients

- ¼ cup lemon juice, freshly squeezed
- 2 tablespoons dill, chopped fresh
- 2 tablespoons sugar, granulated
- 2 tablespoons scallion, finely chopped (green part only)
- ¼ cup of heavy cream
- 1 cucumber, sliced thin
- ¼ teaspoon of freshly ground black pepper
- 2 cups green cabbage, shredded

Directions:

- Mix the cream, sugar, lemon juice, dill, scallion, and pepper in a small bowl until well combined.
- Combine the cabbage and cucumber in a large bowl.
- The salad should be chilled for an hour in the refrigerator.
- Before serving, stir.

Nutritional facts:

- Calories 99

- Fat: 6g
- Carbs: 13g
- Protein: 2g

4.17   Chinese-style turkey salad

- Preparation time: 10 minutes
- Cooking time: 5 minutes
- Serving: 8

Ingredients

- 3 tablespoons canola oil, divided
- 2 tablespoons sesame seeds
- 2 cups turkey, cooked and diced
- 1 green onions, diced
- ½ head cabbage, shredded and chopped
- ¼ cup sugar
- 1 tablespoon vegetable oil
- ½ cup (white) wine vinegar
- 2 packages of ramen noodles

Directions:

- Over medium heat, add 1 tablespoon of canola oil to the skillet.
- When the oil is hot, add the dry noodles and sesame seeds without seasoning, and toast until the noodles become golden brown.
- Stir together the turkey, cabbage, green onion, and cabbage in a bowl.
- The turkey mixture should now include the noodle mixture.

- In another bowl, combine vinegar and 2 tablespoons of canola oil, vegetable oil, and sugar.
- Toss the turkey salad with the vegetable oil dressing until evenly coated.

Nutritional facts:

- Calories 203
- Fat: 6g
- Carbs: 13g
- Protein: 19g

4.18   Watercress and pear salad

- Preparation time: 10 minutes
- Cooking time: 0 minutes
- Serving: 4

Ingredients

- ¼ cup (sweet) onion, coarsely chopped
- 2 pears, cut into wedges
- 1 teaspoon of Dijon mustard
- 1 tablespoon (white) wine vinegar
- 1 teaspoon of honey
- 2 tablespoons olive oil, extra-virgin
- 1 bunch of watercress, remove thick stems, well-washed
- 1 ounce of feta cheese, crumbled

Directions:

- Combine the mustard, onion, vinegar, olive oil, and honey in a blender or food processor until smooth, process.
- Mix the dressing and watercress in a medium bowl. On

four plates, arrange. Add feta cheese crumbles and slices of pear to each.

Nutritional facts:

- Calories 144
- Fat: 8g
- Carbs: 17g
- Protein: 3g

4.19   Salad of roasted beets

- Preparation time: 10 minutes
- Cooking time: 30 minutes
- Serving: 4

Ingredients

- 8 (small) beets, trimmed
- 1 tablespoon (white) wine vinegar
- 2 tablespoons + 1 teaspoon olive oil, extra-virgin, divided
- 1 teaspoon of Dijon mustard
- 4 cups (baby) salad greens
- 2 tablespoons feta cheese, crumbled
- ½ onion, sliced
- 2 tablespoons of walnut pieces
- Freshly ground black pepper

Directions:

- Set the oven's temperature to 400 °F.
- Cook the beets for 30 min, until they are fork-tender, after tossing them with 1 tsp of olive oil and wrapping them in aluminum foil.

- Whisk the other 2 tbsp of olive oil, mustard, and vinegar in a small bowl. Add pepper for flavor.
- Combine the salad leaves, feta cheese, onion, and walnuts in a medium bowl. Toss with approximately one-half of the vinaigrette. Set up on four plates.
- Salads can be topped with sliced beets. Serve with the remaining dressing.

Nutritional facts:

- Calories 170
- Fat: 9g
- Carbs: 20g
- Protein: 4g

4.20   Arugula and celery salad

- Preparation time: 10 minutes
- Cooking time: 0 minutes
- Serving: 4

Ingredients

- 1 shallot, thinly sliced
- 2 cups arugula, loosely packed
- 3 celery stalks, cut into (1-inch) pieces about (¼ inch) thick
- 1 tablespoon olive oil, extra-virgin
- 2 tablespoons Parmesan cheese, grated
- 2 tablespoons (white) wine vinegar
- Freshly ground black pepper

Directions:

- Toss the arugula, celery stalks, and shallot in a medium

bowl.

- ○ Mix the pepper, vinegar, and olive oil in a small bowl. Toss the salad with the dressing after pouring it over it. Add Parmesan cheese on top and serve.

Nutritional facts:

- ○ Calories 45
- ○ Fat: 4g
- ○ Carbs: 1g
- ○ Protein: 1g

Chapter 5: Vegetarian and vegan entrées

What you consume—as well as how much—can have an impact on your health if you have renal disease. You will discover vegan and vegetarian recipes in this chapter that can help you stay healthy and follow a diet that is kind to your kidneys.

<u>5.1</u>   <u>Spicy broccoli and tofu stir-fry</u>

- ◦ Preparation time: 15 minutes
- ◦ Cooking time: 15 minutes
- ◦ Serving: 4

Ingredients
For the sauce

- ◦ 2 tablespoons olive oil, extra-virgin
- ◦ 3 cloves garlic
- ◦ 2 tablespoons of honey
- ◦ 2-inch piece of ginger, peeled
- ◦ ¼ cup rice-wine vinegar

For the stir-fry

- ◦ 1 package (14-ounce) tofu, extra-firm
- ◦ 2 tablespoons olive oil, extra-virgin
- ◦ 1 cup carrots, shredded
- ◦ 2 cups broccoli, chopped
- ◦ 3 scallions, thinly chopped
- ◦ 1 cup white rice, long-grain

Directions:

- ◦ To make the sauce: Combine the garlic, ginger, honey,

vinegar, and olive oil in a food processor, and puree until smooth.

- ○ To make the stir-fry: Cut the tofu into small cubes and press the excess moisture from the tofu using paper towels, repeating several times until dry.
- ○ In a medium pot, cook the rice according to the package directions.
- ○ In a large skillet over medium heat, heat the olive oil. Add the tofu to the pan in a single layer. Carefully add one-quarter of the sauce to the pan and continue to cook, flipping the tofu only once or twice every 4 minutes until it is well browned. With a slotted spoon, transfer the tofu to a plate lined with paper towels to drain.
- ○ Add the broccoli to the pan. Cook, covered, often stirring, until fork-tender, about 5 minutes. Add the carrots and continue to cook for an additional 3 minutes until softened. Add the remaining sauce to the vegetables, return the tofu to the pan, and stir to mix. Garnish with scallions and serve over rice.

Nutritional facts:
- ○ Calories 410
- ○ Fat: 18g
- ○ Carbs: 51g
- ○ Protein: 13g

5.2 Rice and collard-filled red peppers

- ○ Preparation time: 10 minutes
- ○ Cooking time: 50 minutes
- ○ Serving: 4

Ingredients

- 2 medium (red) bell peppers
- ½ onion, chopped
- 2 tablespoons olive oil, extra-virgin, divided
- 6 cups collard greens (loosely packed), trimmed
- 3 cloves garlic, minced
- 1 lemon juice
- 1 cup white rice, cooked
- ¼ cup sunflower seeds, toasted and divided
- Freshly ground black pepper

Directions:

- Set the oven's temperature to 400 °F.
- Remove the stems and seeds from the peppers, then cut them in half lengthwise. Pepper should be sprinkled inside and out of the peppers after 1 tbsp of olive oil has been applied. Put the peppers in a baking tray with the cut side up. Bake for 10 - 15 minutes. After taking the peppers out of the oven, turn them cut side up. Leaving the oven on, set it aside.
- Boil 4 cups of water in a big pot. Cook the collard greens for 5 to 7 minutes or until they are just soft. Drain and then run a cold-water rinse. Slice finely.
- The final tbsp of olive oil should be warmed up in a sizable skillet over medium heat. When the onion is added, sauté it for 5 - 7 minutes, frequently stirring, until it starts to brown. Cook the garlic until aromatic after adding it. Add the collard greens and stir. Stir in the lemon juice and rice after turning the heat off. Use pepper to season.
- Place one tbsp of the sunflower seeds on top of each

pepper half after dividing the mixture among the pepper halves. The baking dish should be filled with 1/4 cup of water, covered with aluminum foil, and heated thoroughly in the oven for 20 minutes. Bake uncovered for a further five minutes.

Nutritional facts:
- Calories 304
- Fat: 9g
- Carbs: 50g
- Protein: 8g

5.3   **Vegan white bean burgers**

- Preparation time: 10 minutes
- Cooking time: 15 minutes
- Serving: 4

Ingredients
- 1 large egg
- 2 teaspoons olive oil, extra-virgin
- 1 cup white beans, canned, drained, and rinsed
- 1 teaspoon powdered garlic
- 1 cup white rice, cooked
- 2 teaspoons thyme, dried
- ½ teaspoon chipotle pepper, ground
- ½ cup corn, fresh/frozen
- ½ onion, finely chopped
- ½ cup (red) bell pepper, finely chopped
- 1 cup of all-purpose flour

- ○ 1 lemon juice
- ○ Freshly ground black pepper

Directions:

- ○ Use a potato masher to thoroughly mash the beans in a big bowl, leaving some whole beans if you like. Mix everything thoroughly before adding the rice, thyme, onion, corn, chipotle pepper, bell pepper, garlic powder, lemon, flour, and egg. Use pepper to season.
- ○ Make four patties out of the mixture using your hands.
- ○ The olive oil should be warmed in a sizable skillet over medium heat. The burgers should be cooked for 5 minutes on one side until browned, then flipped over and cooked for an extra 5 minutes.

Nutritional facts:

- ○ Calories 305
- ○ Fat: 4g
- ○ Carbs: 57g
- ○ Protein: 11g

<u>5.4</u> <u>Strata of red peppers</u>

- ○ Preparation time: 20 minutes
- ○ Cooking time: 1 hour and 5 minutes
- ○ Serving: 4

Ingredients

- ○ 6 eggs
- ○ Butter, for greasing
- ○ 1 tablespoon butter, unsalted

- ½ onion, chopped
- 1 teaspoon garlic, minced
- 1 (red) bell pepper, chopped and boiled
- 1 cup of rice milk
- ¼ cup of tarragon vinegar
- 1 teaspoon of tabasco sauce
- 1-ounce parmesan cheese, grated
- ½ teaspoon of freshly ground black pepper
- 8 slices of white bread, cubes

Directions:

- Set the oven's temperature to 250 °F.
- Butter an ovenproof dish that measures 9 by 9 inches and set it aside.
- Bread cubes should be placed on a baking pan that has been lined with parchment paper.
- The bread cubes should be crisp after 10 minutes in the oven.
- Bread cubes should be taken out of the oven and put aside.
- Melt the butter over medium-high heat in a medium skillet.
- The garlic and onions should be sautéed for about 3 minutes or until tender.
- Red pepper is added, and the cooking time is increased by 2 minutes.
- In the baking dish, layer half the bread cubes, then top with half the sautéed vegetables.
- Repeat with the other half of the vegetables and bread cubes.

- Whisk the eggs, rice milk, vinegar, spicy sauce, and pepper in a medium bowl.
- In the baking dish, evenly distribute the egg mixture.
- The dish should be covered and refrigerated for at least two hours or overnight soaking.
- Ensure that the strata reach room temperature.
- The oven should be heated to 325°F.
- After around 45 minutes, take the plastic wrap off and bake the food until golden.
- Add cheese to the strata's top and bake for an additional five minutes.
- Serve warm.

Nutritional facts:
- Calories 150
- Fat: 6g
- Carbs: 10g
- Protein: 7g

5.5   Thai-inspired vegetable curry

- Preparation time: 15 minutes
- Cooking time: 45 minutes
- Serving: 4

Ingredients
- ½ eggplant, diced
- 2 teaspoons of olive oil
- ½ onion, diced
- 2 teaspoons fresh ginger, grated

- 2 teaspoons garlic, minced
- 1 carrot, diced
- 1 (red) bell pepper, diced
- 1 teaspoon cumin, ground
- 1 tablespoon Curry Powder
- ½ teaspoon of coriander
- A Pinch of cayenne pepper
- 1 tablespoon of cornstarch
- 1½ cups vegetable stock
- ¼ cup of water

Directions:

- Heat the oil in a sizable stockpot over medium-high heat.
- The garlic, onion, and ginger should be sautéed for three minutes or till they are tender.
- For six more minutes, add the carrots, eggplant, and red pepper and continue to sauté while stirring often.
- Add the vegetable stock, curry powder, coriander, cumin, and cayenne pepper.
- Heat should be turned down after the curry comes to a boil. Cook the curry for 30 minutes or till the vegetables are soft.
- Cornstarch and water should be mixed in a small basin.
- Stirring in the cornstarch mixture will thicken the sauce after about 5 minutes of simmering.

Nutritional facts:

- Calories 100
- Fat: 3g

- Carbs: 9g
- Protein: 1g

5.6 Linguine with roasted red pepper–basil sauce

- Preparation time: 20 minutes
- Cooking time: 20 minutes
- Serving: 4

Ingredients

- 1 teaspoon of olive oil
- 8 ounces linguine, uncooked
- ½ onion, chopped
- 1 teaspoon of balsamic vinegar
- 2 teaspoons garlic, minced
- 1 cup red bell peppers, chopped roasted
- ¼ cup fresh basil, shredded
- Freshly ground black pepper
- A Pinch of red pepper flakes
- 4 teaspoons Parmesan cheese (low-fat), grated for garnish

Directions:

- Cook the pasta according to the package instructions.
- While the pasta is cooking, place a large skillet over medium-high heat and add the olive oil.

  Sauté the onions and garlic for about 3 minutes or until they are softened.
- Add the red pepper, vinegar, basil, and red pepper flakes
- to the skillet and stir for about 5 minutes or until heated

through.

- ○ Toss the cooked pasta with the sauce and season with pepper.
- ○ Serve topped with Parmesan cheese.

Nutritional facts:

- ○ Calories 246
- ○ Fat: 3g
- ○ Carbs: 41g
- ○ Protein: 13g

<u>5.7</u>   <u>Mie Goreng with broccoli</u>

- ○ Preparation time: 10 minutes
- ○ Cooking time: 20 minutes
- ○ Serving: 4

Ingredients

- ○ ½ pound of rice noodles
- ○ 2 teaspoons garlic, minced
- ○ ¼ cup dark brown sugar, packed
- ○ 1 teaspoon soy sauce, low sodium
- ○ 1 teaspoon ginger, grated fresh
- ○ ½ teaspoon of sambal oelek
- ○ 1 tablespoon of cornstarch
- ○ 4 ounces (extra-firm) tofu, cubes
- ○ 2 tablespoons of olive oil, divided
- ○ 2 scallions, both (green and white) parts, thinly sliced across the diagonal
- ○ 2 cups broccoli, florets

- ○ Lime wedges for garnish

Directions:

- ○ Cook the noodles according to the package instructions; drain and set aside.
- ○ In a small bowl, whisk together the brown sugar, garlic, ginger, soy sauce, and sambal oelek; set aside.
- ○ Drain the tofu on paper towels for 30 minutes and pat the tofu dry.
- ○ Toss the tofu with the cornstarch and shake to remove the excess.
- ○ In a large skillet over medium-high heat, heat 1 tablespoon of olive oil.
- ○ Add the tofu and sauté for about 10 minutes or until the tofu is browned on all sides and crispy.
- ○ Transfer the tofu to a plate with a slotted spoon.
- ○ Add the remaining 1 tablespoon of oil to the skillet.
- ○ Sauté the broccoli for about 4 minutes or until it is tender.
- ○ Add the sauce and tofu to the skillet and cook for about 2 minutes or until the sauce thickens.
- ○ Serve topped with scallions and garnish with lime wedges.

Nutritional facts:

- ○ Calories 360
- ○ Fat: 11g
- ○ Carbs: 62g
- ○ Protein: 4g

5.8   Fried rice with vegetables

- ○ Preparation time: 20 minutes

- Cooking time: 20 minutes
- Serving: 6

Ingredients

- 3 cups rice, cooked
- 1 tablespoon of olive oil
- ½ onion, chopped
- 2 teaspoons garlic, minced
- ½ cup eggplant, chopped
- 1 cup carrots, sliced
- ½ cup of green beans, cut into (1-inch) pieces
- ½ cup of peas
- 1 tablespoon fresh ginger, grated
- 2 tablespoons fresh cilantro, chopped

Directions:

- In a large skillet over medium-high heat, heat the olive oil.
- Sauté the onion, ginger, and garlic for about 3 minutes or until softened.
- Stir in the carrot, eggplant, peas, and green beans and sauté for 3 minutes more.
- Add the cilantro and rice.
- Sauté, constantly stirring, for about 10 minutes or until the rice is heated through.
- Serve immediately.

Nutritional facts:

- Calories 189
- Fat: 7g

- ○ Carbs: 28g
- ○ Protein: 6g

5.9   **Penne and egg white frittata**

- ○ Preparation time: 15 minutes
- ○ Cooking time: 30 minutes
- ○ Serving: 4

Ingredients

- ○ 6 egg whites
- ○ ¼ cup of rice milk
- ○ 1 tablespoon parsley, chopped fresh
- ○ 2 teaspoons of olive oil
- ○ 1 teaspoon thyme, chopped fresh
- ○ 1 teaspoon chives, chopped fresh
- ○ ¼ (small) onion, chopped
- ○ ½ cup red bell pepper, boiled and chopped
- ○ 1 teaspoon garlic, minced
- ○ 2 cups of cooked penne
- ○ Freshly ground black pepper

Directions:

- ○ Set the oven's temperature to 350 °F.
- ○ Mix the egg whites, parsley, chives, rice milk, thyme, and pepper in a sizable bowl.
- ○ Heat the olive oil over medium heat in a sizable ovenproof skillet.
- ○ The garlic, onion, and red pepper should be softened after 4 minutes of sautéing.

- The cooked penne should be added to the skillet and spread out with a spatula.
- Coat the pasta with the egg mixture by pouring it over the pan and shaking it.
- After one minute, to allow the frittata's bottom to solidify, remove the skillet from the heat and place it in the oven.
- The frittata should bake for about 25 minutes or until it is golden brown and set.
- Take the dish straight out of the oven and serve.

Nutritional facts:
- Calories 170
- Fat: 3g
- Carbs: 25g
- Protein: 10g

<u>5.10 Stuffed spaghetti squash with bulgur</u>

- Preparation time: 20 minutes
- Cooking time: 50 minutes
- Serving: 4

Ingredients

For the squash
- 1 teaspoon of olive oil
- 2 small spaghetti squash, halved
- Freshly ground black pepper

For the filling
- 1 teaspoon of olive oil
- 1 teaspoon garlic, minced

- ½ small onion, finely diced
- ½ cup carrot, chopped
- 1 teaspoon thyme, chopped fresh
- ½ cup of cranberries
- ½ teaspoon cumin, ground
- ½ lemon juice
- ½ teaspoon coriander, ground
- 1 cup bulgur, cooked

Directions:

- For preparing the squash: set the oven's temperature to 350 °F.
- Use parchment paper to cover a baking sheet.
- The sliced sides of the squash should be lightly oiled, seasoned with pepper, and placed cut side down on a baking sheet.
- Bake until soft, about 25 to 30 minutes. Shut off the oven, then turn the squash over in each half.
- Each half should have its flesh removed, leaving the skin on and a 1/2-inch border around the edges.
- In a large bowl, add 2 cups of the squash flesh; save the remaining 2 cups for another purpose.
- For the filling: the olive oil should be heated in a wide skillet on medium heat.
- The cranberries, onion, and carrot should be sautéed for about 6 minutes or until they have softened slightly.
- Squash in the bowl should be combined with the sautéed vegetables.
- Stirring to mix, add the cumin, thyme, and coriander.
- Cooked bulgur and lemon juice should be thoroughly

combined.

- o Fill the squash halves evenly with the filling.
- o Bake for roughly 15 minutes or until thoroughly heated.
- o Serve hot.

Nutritional facts:

- o Calories 111
- o Fat: 2g
- o Carbs: 17g
- o Protein: 3g

5.11 <u>Egg and kale on bread</u>

- o Preparation time: 10 minutes
- o Cooking time: 0 minutes
- o Serving: 2

Ingredients

- o 2 small eggs
- o 2 medium kale leaves
- o ½ teaspoon of olive oil
- o teaspoons (unsalted) butter, divided
- o 2 teaspoons of cream cheese
- o 2 slices of white bread
- o A Pinch of red pepper flakes
- o Freshly ground black pepper

Directions:

- o Preheat the oven to 350°F.
- o Massage the kale leaves with olive oil until they are

completely coated.

- Sprinkle a pinch of red pepper flakes over the kale leaves.
- Place the leaves on a pie plate and roast for about 10 minutes or until crispy.
- Remove the kale from the oven; set aside.
- Butter both sides of the bread with 1 teaspoon of butter per slice.
- In a large skillet over medium-high heat, toast the bread on both sides for about 3 minutes or until it is golden brown.
- Remove the bread from the skillet and spread 1 teaspoon of cream cheese on each slice.
- Melt the remaining 2 teaspoons of butter in the skillet and fry the eggs sunny side up for about 4 minutes.
- Place a piece of crispy kale and a fried egg on top of each slice of the cream cheese–topped bread.
- Serve seasoned with pepper.

Nutritional facts:
- Calories 224
- Fat: 15g
- Carbs: 14g
- Protein: 8g

5.12   Mac and cheese

- Preparation time: 10 minutes
- Cooking time: 25 minutes
- Serving: 4

Ingredients

- 1 teaspoon of olive oil
- Butter, for greasing
- 1 teaspoon garlic, minced
- ½ sweet onion, chopped
- ¼ cup of rice milk
- ½ teaspoon mustard
- 1 cup of cream cheese
- ½ teaspoon of freshly ground black pepper
- 3 cups macaroni, cooked
- A Pinch of cayenne pepper

Directions:

- Turn the oven on to 375°F.
- Butter should be used to grease a 9 by 9-inch baking dish.
- The olive oil should be heated in a wide saucepan on medium heat.
- The garlic and onion should be sautéed for about 3 minutes or until tender.
- Until the mixture is smooth and thoroughly combined, stir in the milk, mustard, cheese, black pepper, and cayenne pepper.
- Stir in the cooked macaroni after adding it.
- Place the baking dish with the mixture inside it in the oven.
- Bake the macaroni for approximately 15 minutes or until bubbling.

Nutritional facts:

- Calories 386
- Fat: 22g

- ○ Carbs: 33g
- ○ Protein: 10g

5.13   <u>Eggplant and tofu stir-fry</u>

- ○ Preparation time: 20 minutes
- ○ Cooking time: 20 minutes
- ○ Serving: 4

Ingredients

- ○ 1 lime juice
- ○ 1 tablespoon sugar, granulated
- ○ 1 tablespoon of all-purpose flour
- ○ 1 teaspoon garlic, minced
- ○ 1 teaspoon ginger, grated fresh
- ○ 1 teaspoon jalapeño pepper, minced
- ○ Water
- ○ 2 cups eggplant, cubed
- ○ 2 tablespoons of olive oil, divided
- ○ 3 tablespoons cilantro, chopped
- ○ 2 scallions, both (green and white) parts, sliced
- ○ 1 ounce of tofu, extra-firm, cut into (½-inch) cubes

Directions:

- ○ Mix the sugar, ginger, flour, garlic, jalapenos, lime juice, and just enough water to form 2/3 cup of sauce in a small bowl; put aside.
- ○ Heat 1 tbsp of the oil in a big skillet on medium heat.
- ○ The tofu should be crisp and brown after 6 minutes in the pan.

- Take out the tofu and place it on a platter.
- The eggplant cubes should be cooked through and faintly browned after about 10 minutes of sautéing in the remaining 1 tbsp oil.
- Toss the tofu, scallions, and other ingredients together in the skillet.
- Pour the sauce in and heat it through while stirring continually for two minutes or until it thickens.
- Before serving, add the cilantro.

Nutritional facts:
- Calories 296
- Fat: 25g
- Carbs: 39g
- Protein: 12g

5.14 Vegetable Biryani

- Preparation time: 10 minutes
- Cooking time: 30 minutes
- Serving: 4

Ingredients
- 1 carrot, diced
- ½ onion, chopped
- 1 cup of basmati rice
- 2 tablespoons olive oil/butter, divided
- ½ teaspoon of cumin seeds
- ½ teaspoon of curry powder
- ½ teaspoon of coriander seeds

- 1 ¾ cups water, divided
- 2 cloves garlic, minced
- 1 teaspoon coriander, ground
- ½ teaspoon cardamom, ground
- ½ teaspoon cumin, ground
- 2 cups of cauliflower florets
- ¼ teaspoon turmeric, ground
- 1 cup of green beans, cut into (2-inch) segments
- ¼ cup cilantro leaves, chopped (for garnish)

Directions:

- Rice should be rinsed in a small bowl until the water is clear. Drain then set apart.
- Heat 1 tbsp of olive oil in a wide stock pot on medium heat.
- Stir continuously for about 30 seconds as you add the cumin seeds, curry powder, and coriander seeds until fragrant. 134 cups of water and rice should both be added to the pot. Boil for a few minutes, then turn the heat down, cover the pot, and cook for 12 minutes. After turning off the heat, let the steam sit covered for 10 min.
- The final tablespoon of olive oil should be heated in a sizable skillet over medium heat. When the onion is soft, add it and simmer for 6 - 8 more minutes. Cook the garlic for one more minute after adding it. Stirring continually, add the turmeric, coriander, cardamom, and cumin to the skillet. Toast for approximately a minute until aromatic. Cook for two to three minutes after adding the beans, cauliflower, and carrots while stirring to coat. Cover the pan with the remaining cup of water and cook for 7 - 10 minutes or till the vegetables are fork-tender.

- Vegetables and rice should be combined by stirring. Serve with cilantro leaves on top.

Nutritional facts:
- Calories 172
- Fat: 4g
- Carbs: 31g
- Protein: 4g

5.15   Pesto cream pasta
- Preparation time: 10 minutes
- Cooking time: 10 minutes
- Serving: 4

Ingredients
- ¼ cup olive oil, extra-virgin
- 8 ounces of linguine noodles
- 2 cups arugula leaves, packed
- 1 cup of walnut pieces
- 2 cups basil leaves, packed
- 3 cloves garlic
- Freshly ground black pepper

Directions:
- Bring the water in a medium stock pot to a boil after filling it halfway. Drain the al dente noodles after cooking.
- Add the basil, walnuts, arugula, and garlic to a food processor. The mixture is coarsely ground. Slowly pour in the olive oil while the food processor is running and blend until creamy. Use pepper to season.

- Combine the pesto with the noodles before serving.

Nutritional facts:
- Calories 394
- Fat: 21g
- Carbs: 0g
- Protein: 10g

5.16 <u>Bowl of roasted vegetables and barley</u>
- Preparation time: 10 minutes
- Cooking time: 30 minutes
- Serving: 4

Ingredients
- 2 small eggplants, diced
- 2 tablespoons olive oil, extra-virgin, divided
- ½ onion, cut into wedges
- ½ (red) bell pepper, chopped
- 1 lemon juice
- 1 cup of barley
- 3 cloves garlic, minced
- ¼ cup feta cheese, crumbled
- ¼ cup basil leaves, roughly chopped
- 2 cups arugula / mixed (baby) salad greens
- Freshly ground black pepper

Directions:
- Set the oven's temperature to 425 °F.
- Combine the zucchini, bell pepper, eggplant, and onion

with 1 tbsp of olive oil in a medium bowl, then spread the vegetables out on a baking sheet in a single layer. Use pepper to season.

- ○ Roast the vegetables, tossing once or twice, for around 25 minutes till they are soft and browned. Leave it alone.
- ○ Add 2 cups water and barley to a medium pot in the meantime. Bring it to a boil, then reduce it to low heat, cover, and simmer for about 20 minutes.
- ○ Take the heat off and give it ten minutes to rest. Drain any additional water before fluffing with a fork.
- ○ Mix the garlic, lemon juice last tbsp of olive oil in a small bowl.
- ○ Combine the barley and veggies in a bowl before adding the lemon-garlic dressing. Add the feta cheese, basil, and salad greens just before serving.

Nutritional facts:
- ○ Calories 292
- ○ Fat: 10g
- ○ Carbs: 44g
- ○ Protein: 9g

<u>5.17 Bulgur and vegetables loaded delicata squash boats</u>

- ○ Preparation time: 10 minutes
- ○ Cooking time: 35 minutes
- ○ Serving: 4

Ingredients
- ○ 6 teaspoons olive oil, extra-virgin divided

- 2 small delicata squash, halved lengthwise and seeded
- ½ onion, diced
- 1 cup of bulgur
- 1 cup black beans, canned, drained, and rinsed
- 2 tablespoons of chili powder
- 2 scallions, thinly sliced (for garnish)
- ½ cup corn kernels, frozen/fresh

Directions:

- Set the oven's temperature to 425 °F.
- Brush the squash pieces with 2 teaspoons olive oil and arrange them on a baking sheet with cut-side down. The flesh should be soft after 20 - 30 minutes of cooking. The 2 cups water and bulgur should be brought to a boil in a separate saucepan. Turn down the heat, cover the pan, and cook for 12 - 15 minutes or till the liquid is dissolved. Drain thoroughly.
- The remaining 4 tsp of olive oil should be heated to medium heat in a large skillet. The onion should only begin to color after 4 - 5 minutes of cooking. Add the corn, black beans, and chili powder after stirring. After adding the bulgur, simmer for another minute.
- Serve the squash halves with the filling divided between them, with scallions on top.

Nutritional facts:

- Calories 314
- Fat: 8g
  Carbs: 56g
- Protein: 10g

<u>5.18</u>   <u>Falafel spinach wrap</u>

- Preparation time: 10 minutes
- Cooking time: 15 minutes
- Serving: 4

Ingredients

- 2 teaspoons cumin, ground
- 6 ounces (baby) spinach
- ¾ cup of flour
- ¼ cup yogurt, plain, unsweetened
- 2 tablespoons of canola oil divided
- 1 can (15-ounce) chickpeas, drained and washed
- 2 cloves garlic, minced
- 1 lemon juice
- 2 red onions, slices
- 1 cucumber, spears
- Salad greens, for serving
- 4 tortillas
- Freshly ground black pepper

Directions:

- Put the spinach in the sink's colander and run boiling water on it to wilt it. After letting it cool, squeeze as much water as you can out of the spinach.
- Add the spinach, cumin, chickpeas, and flour to a food processor. Just blend using a few pulses.
- Utilizing your hands, shape the mixture into tablespoon-sized balls and patties.
- One tablespoon of oil should be heated in a sizable skillet

over medium-high heat. Add one-half of the falafel fattened patties and fry for 2 - 3 minutes per side until golden and crisp. Continue by making additional falafel patties.

○ Mix the yogurt, lemon juice, garlic, and pepper in a small bowl.

○ Put three falafel patties, a few cucumber spears, red onion rings, and salad greens on each tortilla. Add 1 tablespoon of yogurt sauce to the top of each.

Nutritional facts:

○ Calories 241

○ Fat: 17g

○ Carbs: 37g

○ Protein: 8g

5.19   Potato and cauliflower curry

○ Preparation time: 10 minutes

○ Cooking time: 15 minutes

○ Serving: 4

Ingredients

○ 2 tablespoons of canola oil

○ 2-inch piece ginger

○ ½ onion, chopped

○ 3 cloves garlic, minced

○ 1 teaspoon cumin, ground

○ 1 teaspoon turmeric, ground

○ 1 medium-sized potato, diced

○ 1 small green chili, diced

- 1 small cauliflower head, florets
- 2 small tomatoes, diced
- ½ lemon juice
- ½ cup of water
- 1 teaspoon of garam masala
- ¼ cup cilantro leaves, chopped
- Rice/bread for serving

Directions:

- The olive oil should be heated in a big pot over medium heat. Add the onion, and while stirring, cook it until it becomes soft.
- Cook the garlic and ginger until aromatic after adding them. Add the cumin and turmeric after that. Add the water, tomatoes, chili, cauliflower, and potatoes. Simmer, then turn the heat down and cover. Cook the cauliflower and potatoes for 25 minutes, stirring periodically, until they are soft.
- Stir garam masala, cilantro, and lemon juice. Serve with bread or rice.

Nutritional facts:

- Calories 241
- Fat: 17g
- Carbs: 37g
- Protein: 8g

5.20 Sweet pepper, onion, and cabbage medley

- Preparation time: 10 minutes
- Cooking time: 15 minutes

- Serving: 1

Ingredients

- 1 tablespoon of canola oil
- ½ cup (red) bell pepper
- ½ cup (yellow) bell pepper
- ½ cup (green) bell pepper
- ½ cup onions, chopped
- 3 tablespoons of white vinegar
- 2 cups cabbage, shredded
- 1½ teaspoons of brown sugar
- 1½ teaspoons pepper
- 1½ teaspoons of Dijon mustard

Directions:

- Cut the bell peppers into thin strips that are 2 inches long.
- Mix onions, bell peppers, and cabbage together gently in a large nonstick skillet.
- In a jar, combine the vinegar and the remaining ingredients. Secure the lid and shake vigorously.
- Add the veggie mixture while gently stirring.
- Stirring occasionally, sauté the cabbage over medium heat till it becomes soft.

Nutritional facts:

- Calories 70
- Fat: 4g
- Carbs: 8g
- Protein: 1g

Chapter 6: Snacks, condiments, and sides

Even though they occasionally receive a poor rap, snacking can nevertheless play a significant role in your nutrition. A great way to manage hunger between meals is to eat wholesome, delectable snacks. This will also help you choose healthier meals. This chapter contains a good selection of appetizers, sauces, and sides.

6.1 Delicious popcorn

- ◇ Preparation time: 2 minutes
- ◇ Cooking time: 3 minutes
- ◇ Serving: 3

Ingredients

- ◇ ¼ cup of popcorn kernels
- ◇ 1 teaspoon olive oil
- ◇ 1 paper lunch bag

Directions:

- ◇ Popcorn and olive oil should be combined in a bowl.
- ◇ Put the popcorn mixture inside the bag, and secure it with a fold and a staple.
- ◇ Place the bag in the microwave, then cook it for 3 mins on high.
- ◇ Serve and savor.

Nutritional facts:

- ◇ Calories 155
- ◇ Fat: 2g
- ◇ Carbs: 27g

- ◦ Protein: 4g

6.2   <u>Raspberry cream nibbles</u>

- ◦ Preparation time: 10 minutes
- ◦ Cooking time: 0 minutes
- ◦ Serving: 3

Ingredients

- ◦ ¼ cup berry-cream cheese spread (mixed), whipped
- ◦ 3 (medium-sized) raspberries, sliced
- ◦ 1/2 crackers, low sodium

Directions:

- ◦ Just enough whipped cream cheese, blueberries, and raspberries should be added to a bowl.
- ◦ Beat the mixture until it has a smooth texture.
- ◦ Each cracker should have 1 teaspoon of mixed cream cheese berry spread over it.
- ◦ Put a raspberry piece on top of each spread.

Nutritional facts:

- ◦ Calories 134
- ◦ Fat: 8g
- ◦ Carbs: 12g
- ◦ Protein: 2g

6.3 <u>Baba ganoush</u>

- ◦ Preparation time: 20 minutes
- ◦ Cooking time: 30 minutes
- ◦ Serving: 6

Ingredients

- 1 tablespoon olive oil + extra for brushing
- 2 cloves garlic, halved
- 1 medium eggplant, halved and scored on the cut sides in a crosshatch pattern
- 1 large onion, diced
- 1 teaspoon cumin, ground
- 1 teaspoon coriander, ground
- 1 tablespoon lemon juice
- Freshly ground black pepper

Directions:

- Set the oven's temperature to 400 °F.
- Use parchment paper to line two baking sheets.
- Spread the eggplant halves, cut side down, on a baking sheet that has been brushed with olive oil.
- Combine the onion, garlic, cumin, 1 tbsp of olive oil, and coriander in a small bowl.
- On the other baking sheet, spread the seasoned onions.
- Put the onions and eggplant baking sheets into the oven and roast them separately for 20 and 30 minutes, respectively, until they have reached the desired tenderness and color.
- After taking the vegetables out of the oven, scrape the flesh from the eggplant into a bowl.
- On a chopping board, coarsely chop the onions and garlic; add the eggplant.
- Add pepper and lemon juice after stirring.
- Serve hot or cold.

Nutritional facts:

- Calories 45
- Fat: 2g
- Carbs: 6g
- Protein: 1g

6.4 <u>Spicy and sweet kettle corn</u>

- Preparation time: 1 minute
- Cooking time: 5 minutes
- Serving: 8

Ingredients

- 1 cup of popcorn kernels
- 3 tablespoons olive oil
- ½ cup of brown sugar
- A Pinch of cayenne pepper
- **Directions:**

- Put some popcorn kernels and the olive oil in a big saucepan with a lid and heat it on medium heat.
- Lightly shake the saucepan to cause the popcorn to pop. The remaining kernels and sugar should be added to the saucepan.
- When the kernels are completely popped, shake the pot's lid vigorously while continuing to pop the kernels.
- Popcorn is transferred to a big bowl after the heat source is turned off.
- Serve the popcorn after tossing it with cayenne pepper.

Nutritional facts:

- Calories 186
- Fat: 6g
- Carbs: 30g
- Protein: 3g

6.5 Tortilla chips flavored with cinnamon

- Preparation time: 15 minutes
- Cooking time: 10 minutes
- Serving: 6

Ingredients

- Cooking spray
- teaspoons sugar, granulated
- A pinch of nutmeg, ground
- ½ teaspoon cinnamon, ground
- (6-inch) flour tortillas

Directions:

- Set the oven's temperature to 350 °F.
- Use parchment paper to cover a baking sheet.
- Combine the sugar, nutmeg, and cinnamon in a small bowl.
- The tortillas should be placed on a spotless work surface with a small coating of cooking spray on both sides.
- Each tortilla should have a uniform coating of cinnamon sugar.
- Each tortilla should be cut into 16 wedges, then placed on the baking pan.
- The tortilla wedges should bake for about 10 minutes,

flipping once, until crisp.

- Chips can be stored for up to a week at room temperature in an airtight container after cooling.

Nutritional facts:

- Calories 51
- Fat: 1g
- Carbs: 9g
- Protein: 1g

6.6   Meringue cookies

- Preparation time: 30 minutes
- Cooking time: 30 minutes
- Serving: 24 cookies

Ingredients

- 4 egg whites
- 1 teaspoon of vanilla extract
- 1 cup sugar, granulated
- 1 teaspoon of almond extract

Directions:

- Set the oven's temperature to 300 °F.
- Set aside and line two baking pans with paper.
- The egg whites should be beaten to firm peaks in a sizable stainless-steel dish.
- One tablespoon at a time, add the granulated sugar, beating well to combine after each addition, continuing until all the sugar has been added and the meringue is shiny and thick.

- Vanilla and almond extracts should be beaten in.
- Drop the meringue mixture by the tablespoon onto the prepared baking sheets, leaving a little room between each cookie.
- The cookies should bake for about 30 minutes or until crisp.
- Taking the cookies out of the oven, place them on wire racks to cool.
- The cookies can be kept for up to a week at room temperature in an airtight container.

Nutritional facts:

- Calories 36
- Fat: 0g
- Carbs: 8g
- Protein: 1g

6.7 Antojitos

- Preparation time: 20 minutes
- Cooking time: 0 minutes
- Serving: 8

Ingredients

- 6 ounces of cream cheese
- ¼ cup (red) bell pepper, finely chopped
- ½ scallion (green part only) chopped
- ½ jalapeño pepper, thinly chopped
- ½ teaspoon cumin, ground
- ½ teaspoon powdered chili

- ½ teaspoon coriander, ground
- (8-inch) flour tortillas

Directions:

- Mix the cream cheese, jalapenos, scallions, red bell pepper, coriander, cumin, and chili powder thoroughly in a medium bowl.
- Spread a thin layer of cream cheese mixture over each of the 3 tortillas, leaving a 14-inch border all the way around.
- Each tortilla should be tightly wrapped in plastic wrap and rolled like a jelly roll.
- The rolls should be chilled for about an hour or till they are firm.
- To assemble the tortilla rolls on a plate for serving, cut them into 1-inch pieces.

Nutritional facts:

- Calories 110
- Fat: 8g
- Carbs: 7g
- Protein: 2g

6.8 Red pepper crostini with chicken

- Preparation time: 10 minutes
- Cooking time: 5 minutes
- Serving: 4

Ingredients

- 4 ounces of chicken breast, cooked and shredded
- 2 tablespoons of olive oil

- 4 slices of French bread
- ½ teaspoon garlic, minced
- ½ cup fresh basil, chopped

Directions:

- Set the oven's temperature to 400 °F.
- Use aluminum foil to cover a baking sheet.
- Garlic and olive oil should be combined in a small bowl.
- Spread the mixed olive oil on both sides of the bread slices.
- Put the bread on a baking sheet in the oven and bake for 5 minutes, rotating once, or till both sides are crisp and golden.
- Combine the chicken, red pepper, and basil in a medium bowl.
- Red pepper mixture is spread on each slice of toasted bread before serving.

Nutritional facts:

- Calories 184
- Fat: 8g
- Carbs: 19g
- Protein: 9g

6.9 Rice milk

- Preparation time: 5 minutes
- Cooking time: 0 minutes
- Serving: 4

Ingredients

- 4 cups of water
- 1 cup white rice, long-grain
- ½ teaspoon of vanilla extract (optional)

Directions:

- Toast the rice for about 5 minutes over medium heat in a medium, dry skillet.
- Place the water and rice in a container or bowl. Cover, chill, and soak all night.
- Rice, water, and vanilla (if using) should all be placed in a blender and blend until smooth.
- Pour the milk into a glass container or bowl that has been covered with a fine-mesh strainer. Serve right away, or cover put in the fridge, and serve in three days. Before using, shake.

Nutritional facts:

- Calories 112
- Fat: 0g
- Carbs: 24g
- Protein: 0g

6.10 Cheesy pineapple ball

- Preparation time: 5 minutes
- Cooking time: 0 minutes
- Serving: 24

Ingredients

- 20 ounces (canned) pineapple, crushed
  24 ounces of cream cheese

- ½ teaspoon powdered garlic
- ½ cup (green) bell pepper

Directions:

- Place softened cream cheese in a big mixing bowl.
- Well-drain the pineapple. Chop the bell pepper.
- Mix the ingredients in the bowl after adding them.
- The mixture should be formed into a ball. Wax paper wrap, then chill overnight.

Nutritional facts:

- Calories 95
- Fat: 10g
- Carbs: 4g
- Protein: 2g

6.11   Roasted mint-flavored carrots

- Preparation time: 5 minutes
- Cooking time: 20 minutes
- Serving: 6

Ingredients

- 1 tablespoon olive oil, extra-virgin
- 1-pound carrots, trimmed
- ¼ cup mint, thinly sliced
- Freshly ground black pepper

Directions:

- Set the oven's temperature to 425 °F.
- On a baking sheet with a rim, spread the carrots out

evenly. Drizzle the carrots with olive oil and shake them on the baking sheet to coat. Use pepper to season.

- ◦ Roast, stirring twice during cooking, for 20 minutes or until fork-tender and browned. Add the mint and then serve.

Nutritional facts:

- ◦ Calories 51
- ◦ Fat: 2g
- ◦ Carbs: 7g
- ◦ Protein: 1g

6.12 Lime cilantro vinaigrette

- ◦ Preparation time: 5 minutes
- ◦ Cooking time: 0 minutes
- ◦ Serving: ½ cup

Ingredients

- ◦ 1 lime zest
- ◦ ½ cup cilantro stems and leaves, packed
- ◦ 2 tablespoons lime juice, freshly squeezed
- ◦ ¼ cup olive oil, extra-virgin
- ◦ 2 cloves garlic, minced
- ◦ 2 tablespoons of rice vinegar
- ◦ ¼ teaspoon freshly ground black pepper

Directions:

- ◦ Pure the cilantro, lime zest and juice, olive oil, garlic, rice vinegar, and pepper in a blender or food processor. Use instantly or store in the refrigerator for up to two days in an airtight container.

Nutritional facts:

- Calories 50
- Fat: 5g
- Carbs: 1g
- Protein: 0g

6.13   Balsamic vinaigrette

- Preparation time: 5 minutes
- Cooking time: 0 minutes
- Serving: 1 cup

Ingredients

- ¾ cup olive oil, extra-virgin
- 1 teaspoon of Dijon mustard
- ¼ cup of balsamic vinegar
- ½ teaspoon of freshly ground black pepper

Directions:

- Use a whisk to blend pepper, olive oil, mustard, and balsamic vinegar in a bowl. Cover and store in the refrigerator for up to a week.

Nutritional facts:

- Calories 94
- Fat: 10g
- Carbs: 1g
- Protein: 0g

6.14   Lime blueberry sauce

- Preparation time: 5 minutes
- Cooking time: 0 minutes
- Serving: 8

Ingredients

- 6 ounces blueberries, frozen and slightly thawed
- 1 tablespoon lime juice
- 3 tablespoons sugar, granulated
- 1/2 cup of cold water

Directions:

- Fill an electric blender with all the ingredients.
- Blend the mixture until it has a smooth texture.
- Place aside until required.

Nutritional facts:

- Calories 27
- Fat: 1g
- Carbs: 7g
- Protein: 0g

6.15 Cranberry cabbage

- Preparation time: 5 minutes
- Cooking time: 5 minutes
- Serving: 8

Ingredients

- 1 medium-head red cabbage
- 10 ounces (whole) cranberry berry sauce, canned

- 1 tablespoon of lemon juice
- ¼ teaspoon cloves, ground

Directions:

- Cranberry sauce, lemon juice, and cloves are heated in a big skillet and simmered.
- Melted cranberry sauce and cabbage should be combined thoroughly. The mixture should be brought to a boil before being simmered. Stirring occasionally, and continue cooking the cabbage until it is soft.
- Serve warm.

Nutritional facts:

- Calories 73
- Fat: 0g
- Carbs: 18g
- Protein: 1g

Chapter 7: Recipes for meat and poultry

When we think of the low-potassium diet, we don't think about low-potassium meats. But as we have seen here, few poultry and meat recipes do qualify as being low in potassium.

7.1   <u>Thai curried chicken</u>

- ◇ Preparation time: 15 minutes
- ◇ Cooking time: 15 minutes
- ◇ Serving: 4

Ingredients
For the curry paste

- ◇ 2 teaspoons of coriander seeds
- ◇ 2 dried Thai red chiles
- ◇ 1 lemongrass stalk, minced
- ◇ 4 cloves garlic
- ◇ 1 shallot
- ◇ A piece (2-inch) ginger, thinly sliced
- ◇ 1 teaspoon soy sauce, low sodium
- ◇ ½ cup cilantro, coarsely chopped
- ◇ 2 tablespoons of lime juice

For the curry

- ◇ 1-pound (skinless, boneless) chicken breast, thinly sliced
- ◇ 1 teaspoon of canola oil
- ◇ 1 teaspoon of brown sugar
- ◇ 1 cup of green beans, cut into (2-inch) segments
- ◇ 1 lime juice

- ◦ 1 cup water

Directions:
- ◦ To make the curry paste, put the chiles in a bowl and cover them with hot water. Ten minutes are given for soaking.
- ◦ In the meantime, roast the coriander seeds in a small, dry skillet until aromatic, carefully stirring the pan to avoid scorching them. Put it right away in a food processor.
- ◦ Add the drained chiles, shallot, ginger, garlic, soy sauce, cilantro, and lime juice to the food processor. Add up to 2 tbsp of water as necessary to make a fine paste when grinding. Use right away or put in an airtight container to keep chilled for up to 3 days.
- ◦ Heat the oil in a sizable skillet or wok on medium-high heat to prepare the curry. Add the curry paste and cook for about 30 seconds, constantly stirring, until it smells good. When the chicken breast is nearly browned, add it and stir continually.
- ◦ Add one cup of water along with the beans. Simmer for 5 min or until the veggies are soft and the chicken is thoroughly cooked.
- ◦ Brown sugar and lime juice are used as seasonings. Serve with rice or rice noodles.

Nutritional facts:
- ◦ Calories 149
- ◦ Fat: 3g
- ◦ Carbs: 9g
- ◦ Protein: 25g

7.2 Aromatic chicken and cabbage stir-fry

- Preparation time: 10 minutes
- Cooking time: 10 minutes
- Serving: 4

Ingredients

- 10 ounces (skinless, boneless) chicken breast, thinly sliced
- 1 teaspoon of canola oil
- 3 cups of green cabbage, thinly sliced
- 1 teaspoon ginger, ground
- 1 tablespoon of cornstarch
- ½ teaspoon powdered garlic
- Freshly ground black pepper
- ¼ cup of water

Directions:

- The oil should be heated in a sizable skillet over medium-high heat. Toss in the chicken and heat, frequently stirring, until browned and thoroughly cooked.
- When the cabbage is soft but still crispy and green, add it to the pan and simmer for an additional 2 to 3 minutes.
- Combine the cornstarch, water, ginger, and garlic in a small bowl. Put the mixture into the pan and keep heating for another minute or till the sauce has thickened somewhat. Add pepper to taste.

Nutritional facts:

- Calories 96
- Fat: 2g
- Carbs: 5g

- Protein: 15g

7.3   **Baked chicken with herbs**

- Preparation time: 10 minutes
- Cooking time: 40 minutes
- Serving: 6

Ingredients

- 6 chicken thighs, bone-in
- 4 tablespoons butter
- 4 cloves garlic, minced
- 1 tablespoon parsley, chopped fresh
- 1 tablespoon oregano, chopped fresh
- 1 teaspoon of lemon zest
- ¼ teaspoon of freshly ground black pepper

Directions:

- Set the oven's temperature to 425 °F.
- Put the butter, oregano, parsley, lemon zest, and garlic in a small bowl. Mix well.
- Place the chicken thighs on a baking sheet and gently remove the skin while leaving it in place. Replace the skin over the meat after brushing it with a few tsps of the butter mixture. Use pepper to season.
- Bake for about 40 minutes or until the juices are clear and the skin is crisp. Before serving, allow resting for five minutes.

Nutritional facts:

- Calories 226

- Fat: 17g
- Carbs: 1g
- Protein: 16g

7.4   <u>Sour and sweet meatloaf</u>

- Preparation time: 10 minutes
- Cooking time: 50 minutes
- Serving: 8

Ingredients

- 1 large egg
- 1 pound (95% lean) ground beef
- ½ cup onion, chopped
- 2 tablespoons basil, chopped fresh
- 1 teaspoon parsley, chopped fresh
- 1 teaspoon thyme, chopped fresh
- ¼ teaspoon of freshly ground black pepper
- 1 teaspoon of white vinegar
- 1 tablespoon of brown sugar
- ¼ teaspoon powdered garlic
- ½ cup breadcrumbs

Directions:

- Set the oven's temperature to 350 °F.
- Combine the meat, onion, breadcrumbs, egg, thyme, basil, parsley, and pepper.
- In a 9 by 5-inch loaf pan, press the meat mixture
- Combine the vinegar, brown sugar, and garlic powder in a small bowl.

- Over the meat, evenly distribute the brown sugar mixture.
- The meatloaf should be baked for about 50 minutes or until it is thoroughly done.
- Allow the meatloaf to sit for 10 minutes before draining any excess fat.

Nutritional facts:
- Calories 103
- Fat: 3g
- Carbs: 7g
- Protein: 11g

7.5 Cucumber-cilantro salsa with grilled steak

- Preparation time: 20 minutes
- Cooking time: 15 minutes
- Serving: 4

Ingredients
For the salsa
- ¼ cup red bell pepper, boiled and diced
- 1 cup cucumber, chopped
- 2 tablespoons cilantro, chopped fresh
- 1 scallion, both (green and white) parts, chopped
- 1 lime juice

For the steak
- 4 beef (3-ounce) tenderloin steaks
- 2 tablespoon olive oil
- Freshly ground black pepper

Directions:

- How to make the salsa: Combine the bell pepper, cucumber, cilantro, scallion, and lime juice in a medium bowl; place aside.
- How to make a steak: Set a grill to medium-high heat.
- Remove the steaks from the refrigerator and allow them to thaw.
- Pepper is added after olive oil is applied all over the steaks.
- Steaks should be grilled for around 5 minutes on each side for medium rare.
- If you don't have a grill, broil the stakes for 6 minutes on each side in the oven for medium-rare.
- Give the steaks 10 minutes to rest.
- Serve the steaks with the salsa on top.

Nutritional facts:

- Calories 130
- Fat: 6g
- Carbs: 1g
- Protein: 19g

<u>7.6 **Meatloaf with gravy from mushrooms**</u>

- Preparation time: 10 minutes
- Cooking time: 50 minutes
- Serving: 8

Ingredients

- Nonstick cooking spray
- 1 large egg

- 1 tablespoon + 1 teaspoon olive oil, extra-virgin, divided
- 1 onion, finely chopped
- 1 teaspoon oregano, dried
- 3 cloves garlic, minced
- 1½ pounds beef, lean ground
- 1 package(8-ounce) cremini mushrooms, sliced
- 1 white bread slice, breadcrumbs
- 1 tablespoon of all-purpose flour
- ¼ teaspoon of freshly ground black pepper
- 1 cup beef broth, low sodium

Directions:

- Set the oven's temperature to 350 °F. Apply nonstick cooking spray to a loaf pan.
- Heat 1 tbsp of olive oil in a big skillet over medium heat.
- Add the oregano and mushrooms. While intermittently stirring, cook for 5 minutes. After adding the garlic and onions, simmer for another 5 minutes or until the mushrooms and onion are tender. Take it off the heat. Chop one portion of the mushroom combo into fine pieces before dividing it in half. Set aside the other component.
- Add the beef, breadcrumbs, pepper, and mushroom mixture that has been diced to a medium bowl. Mix well. Place the meat mixture in the loaf pan after shaping it into a loaf. Bake for 45 minutes or until cooked through.
- The remaining 1 tsp of olive oil and the remaining mushroom combination should be heated in a pan over medium-high heat. Add the flour and combine to coat. Add the broth gradually while constantly stirring to prevent any clumps after bringing it to a boil, lowering the heat, and

simmering for five minutes to thicken. Serve the meatloaf slices with the gravy.

Nutritional facts:

- ◦ Calories 280
- ◦ Fat: 20g
- ◦ Carbs: 7g
- ◦ Protein: 17g

7.7 Beef stir-up

- ◦ Preparation time: 10 minutes
- ◦ Cooking time: 10 minutes
- ◦ Serving: 6

Ingredients

- ◦ ½ cup onion, chopped
- ◦ ½ pound (95% lean) beef, ground
- ◦ ¼ cup of Herb Pesto
- ◦ ½ cup cabbage, shredded
- ◦ 6 hamburger buns, only the bottom halves

Directions:

- ◦ The meat and onion should be cooked for around 6 minutes in a big skillet on medium heat.
- ◦ Sauté for three minutes more after adding the cabbage.
- ◦ Heat for one minute after adding the pesto.
- ◦ To serve, open the face, split a hamburger bun in half lengthwise, and place one serving of beef mixture on each.

Nutritional facts:

- Calories 120
- Fat: 3g
- Carbs: 13g
- Protein: 11g

7.8   <u>Asian-style chicken satay</u>

- Preparation time: 15 minutes
- Cooking time: 10 minutes
- Serving: 6

Ingredients

- 12 ounces (boneless, skinless) chicken breast, cut into 12 strips
- 2 limes juice
- 1 tablespoon garlic, minced
- 2 tablespoons of brown sugar
- 2 teaspoons ground cumin

Directions:

- Combine the brown sugar, lime juice, cumin, garlic, and in a large bowl.
- Place the bowl with the chicken strips in the fridge for an hour to marinate.
- Set the grill to medium-high heat.
- Chicken should be taken out of the marinade and threaded onto water-soaked wooden skewers, one strip at a time.
- The chicken should be grilled for around 4 minutes on each side or till the meat is well-cooked but still juicy.

Nutritional facts:

- Calories 78
- Fat: 2g
- Carbs: 4g
- Protein: 12g

7.9   Fettuccine with pork ragu

- Preparation time: 10 minutes
- Cooking time: 30 minutes
- Serving: 6

Ingredients

- 200g pork, ground lean
- 350g fettuccine
- 5 tablespoons of canola oil
- 1 medium-sized zucchini, chopped
- ½ large onion, diced
- 200ml vegetable stock, without salt
- 2 medium (red) peppers, thinly sliced
- 1 garlic clove, finely chopped
- 2 teaspoons truffle oil
- 1/8 teaspoon chili pepper

Directions:

- Large pan on medium heat with canola oil added.
- Sauté the garlic and onion in the pan until they are golden.
- Sauté the garlic combination before adding the minced pork.
- When the pork is well done, raise the heat to medium and

stir-fry for 8 minutes.

- Stir in the zucchini, red pepper, and chili pepper; simmer for approximately 5 minutes or until the vegetables are soft.
- Cook for an additional 8 minutes after adding the vegetable stock to the mixture.

TIP: Be careful not to overdo the sauce to prevent it from becoming dry.

- Over medium heat, add water to a different pan and bring to a boil.
- Pasta should be cooked in boiling water for about 5 minutes or until it reaches the desired texture.
- Add the pasta to the sauce-filled pot after draining.
- The mixture should be thoroughly combined until the sauce is distributed evenly and the pasta seems creamy.

TIP: To moisten pasta, if it seems dry, add a small bit of cooking water.

- Place the pasta mixture on plates and top each one with a teaspoon of truffle oil.

Nutritional facts:

- Calories 458
- Fat: 2g
- Carbs: 31g
- Protein: 16g

7.10 Satay chicken with peanut sauce

Preparation time: 10 minutes
Cooking time: 10 minutes

- Serving: 6

Ingredients

For the chicken

- 1-pound (boneless, skinless) chicken breast, cut into strips
- ½ cup yogurt, unsweetened
- A piece (1-inch) ginger, minced
- 2 cloves garlic, minced
- 2 teaspoons powdered curry
- 1 teaspoon of canola oil

For the peanut sauce

2
- limes juice
- ¾ cup smooth peanut butter, unsalted
- 1 teaspoon of soy sauce
- ½ teaspoon (red) chili flakes
- Cilantro leaves, chopped
- 1 tablespoon brown sugar
- ¼ cup of hot water
- Lime wedges (for garnish)

Directions:

- To prepare the chicken, combine the yogurt, ginger, garlic, and curry powder in a small bowl. Mix by stirring. Chicken strips should be added to the marinade. For two hours, cover and chill.
- Chicken chunks are skewered with thread.
- Heat a grill pan on medium-high after brushing with oil. The chicken skewers should be cooked thoroughly for 3 to 5 minutes on each side.

- The following ingredients are needed to prepare the peanut sauce: peanut butter, brown sugar, soy sauce, lime juice, and boiling water until smooth, process. Add cilantro after transferring to a bowl. Serve the chicken satay with wedges of lime to squeeze over the skewers.

Nutritional facts:
- Calories 458
- Fat: 2g
- Carbs: 31g
- Protein: 16g

Chapter 8: Fish and seafood dishes

Omega-3 fatty acids may improve blood pressure and lower blood fat levels. Considering that lowering blood pressure naturally reduces the chance of renal disease, doing so may aid in safeguarding the kidneys.

8.1   Garlic lemon halibut

- Preparation time: 10 minutes
- Cooking time: 15 minutes
- Serving: 4

Ingredients

- 1 lemon zest
- ¼ cup lemon juice, freshly squeezed
- 2 cloves garlic, minced
- 2 tablespoons olive oil, extra-virgin, divided
- Freshly ground black pepper
- 1 pound of halibut filets, skin removed
- 2 tablespoons parsley, chopped fresh
- 2 tablespoons cilantro, chopped fresh

Directions:

- Set the oven's temperature to 400 °F.
- Combine the lemon juice, garlic, and 1 tbsp of olive oil in a medium bowl. Use pepper to season. Put the halibut filets in and give them a quick spin to coat. Marinate in the refrigerator for 10 minutes.
- Brush the marinade over the filets before placing them on a baking sheet. Cook for 12 – 15 minutes, basting once

halfway through with the marinade. Cook until a fork can easily pierce the fish. Remove the fish from the marinade and top with cilantro, lemon zest, and parsley before serving.

Nutritional facts:
- Calories 169
- Fat: g
- Carbs: 2g
- Protein: 21g

<u>8.2</u>   <u>Shrimp scampi linguine</u>
- Preparation time: 15 minutes
- Cooking time: 15 minutes
- Serving: 4

Ingredients
- 1 lemon juice
- 4 ounces linguine, uncooked
- 1 teaspoon of olive oil
- 4 ounces shrimp, chopped
- 2 teaspoons garlic, minced
- ½ cup white wine, dry
- ½ cup heavy whipped cream
- 1 tablespoon basil, chopped fresh
- Freshly ground black pepper

Directions:
- Follow the directions on the package to cook the linguine, then drain it and set it aside.

- ◦ The olive oil should be warmed in a sizable skillet over medium heat.
- ◦ For about 6 minutes, or till the shrimp is slightly opaque and cooked through, sauté the shrimp and garlic together.
- ◦ Cook for 5 min after adding the lemon juice, wine, and basil.
- ◦ Add the cream and boil for a further two minutes.
- ◦ Toss the linguine in the skillet with the sauce.
- ◦ To serve, divide the spaghetti among 4 dishes.

Nutritional facts:
- ◦ Calories 219
- ◦ Fat: 17g
- ◦ Carbs: 21g
- ◦ Protein: 12g

<u>8.3</u>   <u>Seafood casserole</u>
- ◦ Preparation time: 20 minutes
- ◦ Cooking time: 45 minutes
- ◦ Serving: 6

Ingredients
- ◦ 4 ounces shrimp, cooked
- ◦ 1 large egg
- ◦ 2 cups eggplant, diced into (1-inch) pieces
- ◦ 1 tablespoon of olive oil
- ◦ 1 teaspoon garlic, minced
- ◦ ½ small onion, chopped
- ◦ ½ cup of white rice, uncooked

- 1 stalk of celery, chopped
- 3 tablespoons lemon juice, freshly squeezed
- ½ (red) bell pepper, chopped and boiled
- 1 teaspoon of hot sauce
- ¼ teaspoon of Creole Seasoning Mix
- 6 ounces of crab meat
- Butter, for greasing

Directions:

- Set the oven's temperature to 350°F.
- The eggplant should boil for 5 minutes in a small saucepan of water over medium-high heat. Drain, then place in a big basin.
- A 9 by 13-inch baking dish should be butter-greased and placed aside.
- The olive oil should be warmed in a sizable skillet over medium heat.
- The bell pepper, celery, onion, and garlic should be sautéed for about 4 minutes or until they are soft.
- Add the rice, egg, lemon juice, spicy sauce, creole spice, and sautéed vegetables to the eggplant.
- To blend, stir.
- Add the crab and shrimp after folding.
- Place the casserole ingredients inside the dish and smooth the top.
- Bake the casserole for 25 - 30 minutes, or until the rice is cooked through and the dish is well warm.
- Serve hot.

Nutritional facts:

- Calories 118
- Fat: 4g
- Carbs: 9g
- Protein: 12g

8.4 Haddock baked in an herb crust

- Preparation time: 10 minutes
- Cooking time: 20 minutes
- Serving: 4

Ingredients

- 12-ounce haddock filets, skinned and deboned
- ¼ teaspoon of freshly ground black pepper
- ½ cup breadcrumbs
- 1 tablespoon of lemon zest
- 3 tablespoons parsley, chopped fresh
- 1 teaspoon thyme, chopped fresh
- 1 tablespoon butter, unsalted and melted

Directions:

- Set the oven's temperature to 350 °F.
- The breadcrumbs, lemon zest, parsley, thyme, and pepper should all be thoroughly mixed in a small basin.
- Mix in the melted butter until the material looks like coarse crumbs.
- Haddock should be placed on a baking sheet, and the bread crumb batter should be spooned on top and pressed down firmly.
- Haddock is done when it is opaque throughout and flakes

apart into chunks when pressed after being baked for about 20 minutes.

Nutritional facts:

- Calories 143
- Fat: 3g
- Carbs: 10g
- Protein: 16g

8.5 Herb-pesto tuna

- Preparation time: 10 minutes
- Cooking time: 10 minutes
- Serving: 4

Ingredients

- 4 yellowfin (3-ounce) tuna filets
- 1 teaspoon of olive oil
- 1 lemon, cut into (8 thin) slices
- Freshly ground black pepper
- ¼ cup of Herb Pesto

Directions:

- Set the grill to medium-high heat.
- Sprinkle each piece of fish with pepper and drizzle with olive oil.
- On the grill, cook the fish for 4 minutes.
- After flipping it over, add lemon slices and herb pesto to each piece of fish.
- Grill the tuna for a further 5 to 6 minutes or until it is well done.

Nutritional facts:

- Calories 103
- Fat: 2g
- Carbs: 0g
- Protein: 21g

8.6   <u>Fish with pineapple salsa</u>

- Preparation time: 10 minutes
- Cooking time: 20 minutes
- Serving: 4

Ingredients

For the pineapple salsa

- ½ lime juice
- 1 cup pineapple, diced
- ½ jalapeno pepper, diced
- ¼ cup (red) onion, diced
- ¼ cup cilantro, chopped fresh

For the fish

- 1-pound filets of white fish
- 1 egg, beaten
- 1 tablespoon butter
- ½ teaspoon of paprika
- 2 tablespoons rice milk
- ¼ cup of yellow cornmeal
- ½ teaspoon powdered garlic
- ¼ cup of all-purpose flour

Directions:

For the salsa: Combine the onion, cilantro, lime juice, and jalapeño in a small bowl. Stir and put aside while preparing the fish.

For the fish:

- Set the oven's temperature to 400 °F. Small baking dish with butter.
- The fish filets are seasoned with paprika and garlic powder.
- Cornmeal and flour should be combined in a small bowl.
- Combine the rice milk and egg in a separate small bowl.
- Each filet of fish should be dipped in the egg blend before being rolled into the flour mix. Put the fish in the pan as is, in a single layer. Fish should be golden and flake easily with a fork after 20 minutes of baking, flipping once halfway through.

Nutritional facts:

- Calories 242
- Fat: 7g
- Carbs: 20g
- Protein: 27g

8.7 Kale and Salmon on parchment

- Preparation time: 10 minutes
- Cooking time: 15 minutes
- Serving: 4

Ingredients

- 1 pound salmon filets
- 1 lemon, sliced

- ○ 2 cups kale leaves, thinly sliced
- ○ ½ teaspoon paprika
- ○ 4 thyme sprigs, fresh
- ○ 2 small zucchinis, sliced
- ○ 4 rosemary sprigs
- ○ ¼ cup dry white wine
- ○ Freshly ground black pepper

Directions:

- ○ Set the oven's temperature to 450 °F .
- ○ The diameter of each of the four parchment paper pieces should be roughly 12 inches.
- ○ Place a half-cup of kale leaves and a few slices of zucchini on top of each paper. Use pepper to season.
- ○ The salmon filets are paprika-seasoned, and then a sprig of thyme, a sprig of rosemary, and a lemon slice are placed on top of each filet. Each filet should get 1 tbsp of white wine.
- ○ The parchment paper should be folded over, the seams sealed with a crease.
- ○ For 15 minutes, bake. Before serving, take the filets out of the oven and allow them to cool for around 5 minutes.

Nutritional facts:

- ○ Calories 207
- ○ Fat: 7g
- ○ Carbs: 60g
- ○ Protein: 26g

8.8   Cod with dill - cucumber salsa

- Preparation time: 20 minutes
- Cooking time: 10 minutes
- Serving: 4

Ingredients
For the cucumber salsa

- ¼ cup red bell pepper, boiled and minced
- ½ cucumber, chopped
- 2 tablespoons fresh dill, chopped
- 1 lime zest
- 1 lime juice
- ½ teaspoon sugar, granulated

For the fish

- 12 ounces cod filets, boneless and cut into 4 servings
- 1 teaspoon of olive oil
- ½ teaspoon of freshly ground black pepper
- 1 lemon juice

Directions:

- Cucumber salsa preparation: Combine the cucumber, lime juice, red pepper, dill, lime zest, and sugar in a small bowl; leave aside.
- To prepare the fish, preheat your oven to 350°F.
- On a pie plate, arrange the fish filets and drizzle with the lemon juice.
- Then equally distribute the olive oil and pepper over the filets.
- The fish should be baked for about 6 minutes or until a fork can easily pierce it.

- ○ Serve the fish on 4 plates with cucumber salsa on top.

Nutritional facts:
- ○ Calories 110
- ○ Fat: 2g
- ○ Carbs: 3g
- ○ Protein: 20g

8.9 <u>Grilled shrimp with a lime cucumber salsa</u>

- ○ Preparation time: 15 minutes
- ○ Cooking time: 10 minutes
- ○ Serving: 4

Ingredients
- ○ 6 ounces large shrimp, tails left on
- ○ 2 tablespoons of olive oil
- ○ 1 teaspoon garlic, minced
- ○ ½ cup mango, chopped
- ○ ½ cup cucumber, chopped
- ○ 1 lime juice
- ○ 1 lime zest
- ○ Lime wedges for garnish
- ○ Freshly ground black pepper

Directions:
- ○ Put four wooden skewers in a bowl of water for half an hour.
- ○ Heat the grill to a medium-high setting.
- ○ Mix the shrimp, garlic, and olive oil in a sizable bowl.

- Thread four shrimp on each skewer.
- Combine the cucumber, lime juice, mango, and zest in a small bowl. Sprinkle a little pepper over the salsa before serving. Place aside.
- The shrimp should be cooked through and opaque after grilling for around 10 minutes, rotating once.
- Pepper should be used sparingly on the shrimp.
- Serve the shrimp over the cucumber salsa, with wedges of lime on the side.

Nutritional facts:

- Calories 120
- Fat: 8g
- Carbs: 4g
- Protein: 9g

8.10   Linguine with scampi shrimp

- Preparation time: 15 minutes
- Cooking time: 15 minutes
- Serving: 4

Ingredients

- 1 lemon juice
- 4 ounces linguine, uncooked
- 1 teaspoon of olive oil
- 4 ounces shrimp, chopped
- ½ cup (dry) white wine
- 2 teaspoons garlic, minced
- ½ cup heavy whipped cream

- 1 tablespoon fresh basil, chopped
- Freshly ground black pepper

Directions:

- Linguine should be prepared per the directions on the package. Drain then set aside.
- The olive oil should be warmed in a big skillet over medium heat.
- For about 6 minutes, or till the shrimp is slightly opaque and cooked through, sauté the shrimp and garlic together.
- Add lemon juice, wine, and basil; cook for 5 minutes.
- Add the cream and boil for a further two minutes.
- Mix the linguine with the sauce in the skillet.
- Serve the pasta by dividing it among 4 plates.

Nutritional facts:

- Calories 219
- Fat: 17g
- Carbs: 21g
- Protein: 17g

Chapter 9: Beverages and smoothies recipes

Drink homemade smoothies to increase your consumption of high-quality protein and low-potassium fruit. When days become busy, these simple smoothies and beverages are a quick cure for a healthy snack or dinner replacement.

9.1   Berry-bursting smoothie

- Preparation time: 5 minutes
- Cooking time: 0 minutes
- Serving: 1

Ingredients

- 1 cup blueberries, frozen
- 6 tablespoons of protein powder
- 14 ounces apple juice (without sugar)
- 8 cubes ice
- 8 Splenda packets

Directions:

- In a blender, combine all the ingredients and blend until smooth.

Nutritional facts:

- Calories 108
- Fat: 0g
- Carbs: 18g
- Protein: 9g

9.2   <u>Berries mint water</u>

- ◦ Preparation time: 5 minutes
- ◦ Cooking time: 0 minutes
- ◦ Serving: 8

Ingredients

- ◦ ½ cup strawberries
- ◦ 8 cups of water
- ◦ 3 mint sprigs
- ◦ ½ cup blackberries

Directions:

- ◦ Combine the water, blackberries, strawberries, and mint in a big pitcher; before consuming, cover and refrigerate for at least one hour. Keep in the fridge for no more than two days.

Nutritional facts:

- ◦ Calories 77
- ◦ Fat: 0g
- ◦ Carbs: 2g
- ◦ Protein: 0g

9.3   <u>Chia vanilla smoothie</u>

- ◦ Preparation time: 5 minutes
- ◦ Cooking time: 0 minutes
- ◦ Serving: 2

Ingredients

- ◦ 1 cup rice milk

- 1 teaspoon of honey
- 1 teaspoon of vanilla extract
- ½ teaspoon cinnamon, ground
- 2 tablespoons of chia seeds
- ½ teaspoon ginger, ground
- 2 bags of black tea
- 1 cup of ice
- ¼ teaspoon cloves, ground
- ¼ teaspoon cardamom, ground

Directions:

- Rice milk should be heated to just steaming in a small pan. After five minutes of brewing, discard the tea bags.
- Rice milk, ice, honey, cardamom, vanilla, cinnamon, chia seeds, ginger, and cloves should all be combined in a blender. Blend until smooth, then serve.

Nutritional facts:

- Calories 143
- Fat: 5g
- Carbs: 19g
- Protein: 3g

9.4 Pina colada Smoothie

- Preparation time: 5 minutes
- Cooking time: 0 minutes
- Serving: 2

Ingredients

- ½ cup pineapple (unsweetened) juice

- 1 cup pineapple, canned/fresh
- 1 cup (8 ounces) tofu, firm
- 1/8 teaspoon flakes of red pepper
- 1 teaspoon Stevia /Stevia /another sweetener

Directions:

- In a blender, blend all the ingredients until smooth, and serve.

Nutritional facts:

- Calories 189
- Fat: 3g
- Carbs: 32g
- Protein: 13g

<u>9.5</u> <u>Oat banana shake</u>

- Preparation time: 5 minutes
- Cooking time: 0 minutes
- Serving: 2

Ingredients

- ½ cup oatmeal, cooked and chilled
- 2 tablespoons of brown sugar
- 2/3 cup of skim milk
- 1 ½ teaspoons of vanilla extract
- 1 tablespoon of wheat germ
- ½ banana, chunks

Directions:

- Blend the oatmeal in a blender for a while.

- Pour in the milk, wheat germ, vanilla, and one-half of a banana. Blend until smooth and thick.

Nutritional facts:
- Calories 172
- Fat: 4g
- Carbs: 33g
- Protein: 10g

9.6 Smoothie with strawberry cheesecake

- Preparation time: 5 minutes
- Cooking time: 0 minutes
- Serving: 2

Ingredients
- 1 cup rice milk
- 1 teaspoon of vanilla extract
- 1 cup of strawberries, hulled
- ½ teaspoon of honey
- 2 tablespoons of cream cheese
- 5 cubes of ice

Directions:
- Blend the ice cubes, honey, vanilla, rice milk, and cream cheese in a blender until smooth. Blend until smooth, then serve.

Nutritional facts:
- Calories 114
- Fat: 6g

- Carbs: 13g
- Protein: 1g

9.7   <u>Apple lemon smoothie</u>

- Preparation time: 5 minutes
- Cooking time: 0 minutes
- Serving: 4

Ingredients

- 1 banana
- 1 cup of vanilla yogurt, frozen
- 1 apple, peeled and cored
- 2-3 teaspoons of honey
- ¼ cup lemon juice
- ½ cup apple juice

Directions:

- Use a blender to mix all the ingredients until they are smooth.
- Put in a large, chilled glass.

Nutritional facts:

- Calories 170
- Fat: 0.8g
- Carbs: 37g
- Protein: 5g

9.8   <u>Raspberry peach smoothie</u>

- Preparation time: 5 minutes

- Cooking time: 0 minutes
- Serving: 3

Ingredients

- 1 medium peach, sliced
- 1 cup raspberries, frozen
- 1 tablespoon honey
- ½ cup tofu
- 1 cup almond milk, unfortified

Directions:

- In a blender, blend each ingredient until it is smooth.

Nutritional facts:

- Calories 129
- Fat: 3g
- Carbs: 23g
- Protein: 6g

9.9 Mint Lassi

- Preparation time: 5 minutes
- Cooking time: 0 minutes
- Serving: 2

Ingredients

- 1 teaspoon of cumin seeds
- 1 cup yogurt, unsweetened
- ½ cup mint leaves
- ½ cup of water

Directions:

- Roast the cumin seeds in a dry skillet on medium heat until fragrant, about 1 to 2 minutes.
- Transfer the seeds, mint, yogurt, and water to a blender, and blend until smooth.

Nutritional facts:

- Calories 114
- Fat: 6g
- Carbs: 5g
- Protein: 10g

9.10   <u>Cinnamon horchata</u>

- Preparation time: 5 minutes
- Cooking time: 0 minutes
- Serving: 4

Ingredients

- 1 cup of white rice, long-grain
- 1 cinnamon stick piece
- 4 cups of water
- 1 cup rice milk
- 1 cup sugar, granulated
- 1 teaspoon cinnamon, ground
- 1 teaspoon of vanilla extract

Directions:

- Rice, water, and chunks of the cinnamon stick should all be combined in a blender. The rice should start to break up after about a minute of blending. Allow it to sit for at least three hours or overnight at room temperature.

- Pour the liquid into a pitcher over a wire mesh strainer.
- Throw away the rice.
- Add sugar, milk, vanilla, and ground cinnamon. To blend, stir.
- Serving with ice.

Nutritional facts:

- Calories 123
- Fat: 4g
- Carbs: 26g
- Protein: 1g

9.11   Kiwi watermelon smoothie

- Preparation time: 5 minutes
- Cooking time: 0 minutes
- Serving: 2

Ingredients

- 2 cups of watermelon chunks
- 1 cup of ice
- 1 kiwifruit, peeled

Directions:

- In a blender, combine watermelon, ice, and kiwi, processing until smooth.

Nutritional facts:

- Calories 67
- Fat: 0g

- ◦ Carbs: 17g
- ◦ Protein: 1g

9.12   <u>Digestive cooler fennel</u>

- ◦ Preparation time: 5 minutes
- ◦ Cooking time: 15 minutes
- ◦ Serving: 2

Ingredients

- ◦ ¼ cup of fennel seeds, ground
- ◦ 2 cups of rice milk
- ◦ 1 tablespoon honey
- ◦ ¼ teaspoon cloves, ground

Directions:

- ◦ The milk, cloves, fennel seeds, and honey should all be put in a blender. Once smooth, process again and let sit for 30 minutes.
- ◦ Pour through a coffee filter or cheesecloth-lined wire mesh strainer into a container of your choice. Serve.

Nutritional facts:

- ◦ Calories 163
- ◦ Fat: 2g
- ◦ Carbs: 30g
- ◦ Protein: 3g

9.13   <u>Cranberry and ginger punch</u>

- ◦ Preparation time: 5 minutes
- ◦ Cooking time: 5 minutes

- Serving: 4

Ingredients

- 4 cups of cranberry juice
- 1/3 cup of lime juice
- ½ cup ginger, sliced thin
- 1/3 cup sugar, granulated

Directions:

- In a big pan, boil the juice and ginger.
- Infuse flavor by cooking for about 20 minutes over medium heat.
- Stir until sugar and lime juice are completely dissolved.
- Drain, then serve.

Nutritional facts:

- Calories 124
- Fat: 2g
- Carbs: 31g
- Protein: 6g

9.14 Orange and blueberry-infused water

- Preparation time: 5 minutes
- Cooking time: 0 minutes
- Serving: 6

Ingredients

- ¼ cup of blueberries
- 1 orange
- 1 liter (33 ounces) of filtered water

Directions:

- Put the blueberries in the glass, and then use the back of a spoon to gently crush them up so that their juices can release.
- Oranges should be cut into quarters, and each quarter should be squeezed into a big jug with a lid.
- Mix the water, the slightly mashed blueberries, and the orange quarters in a big jug.
- Put in the refrigerator for a few hours or overnight.
- Drink as soon as possible after making the best results.

Nutritional facts:

- Calories 14
- Fat: 1g
- Carbs: 3g
- Protein: 1g

9.15 Spinach and cucumber smoothie

- Preparation time: 5 minutes
- Cooking time: 0 minutes
- Serving: 2

Ingredients

- ½ green apple, chopped
- ½ cucumber, chopped
- 2 cups of spinach
- 1 cup rice milk
- 3 cubes of ice

Directions:

- Blend the spinach, cucumber, apple, milk, and ice in a blender. Blend until smooth, then serve.

Nutritional facts:

- Calories 75
- Fat: 2g
- Carbs: 14g
- Protein: 1g

Chapter 10: Desserts

When on the kidney diet, some bakery items are off-limits. This does not preclude you from enjoying baked goods. One way to get the fresh-from-the-oven taste you crave while maintaining control over the ingredients is to bake them at home.

10.1   Flavorful shortbread cookies

- Preparation time: 10 minutes
- Cooking time: 15 minutes
- Serving: 16 cookies

Ingredients

- 1 cup of all-purpose flour
- ½ cup (unsalted) butter, cut into (½-inch) cubes
- ½ cup powdered sugar, + extra for shaping cookies
- 1 lemon zest
- 1 lime zest

Directions:

- Turn the oven on to 375°F.
- Add the sugar, flour, butter, and zest of the lime and lemon to a food processor. Just before the dough comes together, process.
- Use your hands to form a ball out of a tablespoon of dough. Roll the dough into balls and put it on a baking pan as you go, using all the dough.
- The balls are pressed flat with the base of a measuring cup that has been dunked in powdered sugar.
- The edges should only be lightly browned after baking for

13 - 15 minutes. A wire rack should be used to cool the cookies. Store for up to five days in an airtight container.

Nutritional facts:

- ◦ Calories 94
- ◦ Fat: 6g
- ◦ Carbs: 10g
- ◦ Protein: 1g

10.2   Tropical granita

- ◦ Preparation time: 10 minutes
- ◦ Cooking time: 0 minutes
- ◦ Serving: 4

Ingredients

- ◦ 1 lime juice
- ◦ 1 cup pineapple chunks, fresh/frozen
- ◦ 2 cups of orange juice
- ◦ ½ cup mango chunks, fresh/frozen
- ◦ Fresh mint, for garnish

Directions:

- ◦ The pineapple, orange juice, mango, and lime juice should all be combined in a blender. Transfer to a dish that can be frozen after processing until smooth. For two hours, freeze.
- ◦ To separate the mixture into more manageable granular pieces, use a fork. Serve with shredded mint leaves as a garnish.

Nutritional facts:

- Calories 103
- Fat: 0g
- Carbs: 26g
- Protein: 1g

10.3   **Apple Dutch pancake**

- Preparation time: 10 minutes
- Cooking time: 30 minutes
- Serving: 8

Ingredients

- 3 eggs
- 2 tablespoons butter, unsalted
- 3 large apples, sliced
- ½ cup of all-purpose flour
- 1 teaspoon cinnamon, ground
- 1 teaspoon lemon zest, grated
- 6 tablespoons sugar, granulated
- ½ cup of milk
- 1 tablespoon of sour cream
- ¼ teaspoon salt

Directions:

- In an oven-safe pan, melt butter on medium-high heat.
- Apples, sugar, and cinnamon added; cook and stir for 3 to 5 minutes. Get rid of the heat.
- Beat eggs in a bowl until foamy. Combine the milk, flour, sour cream, salt, and zest.
- Beat until an even batter is produced.

- Pour over the apples, then bake for 25 minutes at 400 °F until the apples are puffy and golden brown.
- Slice into wedges and serve straight from the skillet.

Nutritional facts:
- Calories 339
- Fat: 11g
- Carbs: 54g
- Protein: 8g

10.4 Grape galette

- Preparation time: 15 minutes
- Cooking time: 25 minutes
- Serving: 6

Ingredients

For the crust
- 4 tablespoons of cold butter, cut into (½-inch) cubes
- 1 cup of all-purpose flour
- ½ cup of rice milk
- 1 tablespoon of sugar

For the galette
- 1 egg white
- 2 cups grapes, halved seedless
- 1 tablespoon of cornstarch
- 1 cup sugar

Directions:
- To prepare the crust, combine the sugar and flour in the

food processor and pulse only a few times to combine. Once the butter has been added, pulse the food several times until a coarse meal appears. When the dough is crumbly, mix the rice milk and knead it together.

- Take the dough and flatten it into a disc on a clean surface. Refrigerate for two hours or overnight after wrapping in plastic wrap.
- Prepare the oven by setting it to 425 °F .
- Mix the cornstarch and sugar in a medium bowl. Grapes are added; toss to combine.
- The dough should be unwrapped and laid out on a floured board. Create a 14-inch circle with it and place it in a cast-iron or other oven-safe skillet.
- Spread the grape filling outward from the middle of the dough, leaving a 2-inch crust border. The dough's borders are folded inward to partially enclose the grapes.
- Use egg white to brush the dough. Cook the crust for 20 - 25 minutes or until brown. Rest 20 mins before serving.

Nutritional facts:

- Calories 172
- Fat: 6g
- Carbs: 27g
- Protein: 2g

10.5 Raspberry mousse cheesecake

- Preparation time: 15 minutes
- Cooking time: 0 minutes
- Serving: 6

Ingredients

- 1 package (8 ounces) of cream cheese
- 1 cup light whipped topping
- ¾ cup sweetener, granular with no calorie
- 1 teaspoon vanilla extract
- 1 teaspoon lemon zest, finely grated
- 1 cup raspberries, fresh/frozen

Directions:

Cream cheese should be creamy before adding 1/2 cup of Granular sweetener and beating until it is melted. Vanilla and lemon zest are combined.

Put a few raspberries aside for decoration. With a fork, mash the remaining raspberries, then toss in the remaining 1/4 cup of Granular sweetener until it has melted.

Gently but quickly incorporate the crushed raspberries after folding in the light whipped topping to the cream cheese mixture.

The mousse should be divided among six glasses and chilled until serving time.

Serve mousse with a garnish of mint and fresh raspberries.

Nutritional facts:

- Calories 257
- Fat: 15g
- Carbs: 29g
- Protein: 3g

<u>10.6</u>   <u>Meringue almond cookies</u>

- Preparation time: 15 minutes
- Cooking time: 25 minutes
- Serving: 24 small cookies

Ingredients

- 2 eggs
- ½ teaspoon vanilla extract
- 1 teaspoon cream of tartar
- ½ cup of white sugar
- ½ teaspoon almond extract

Directions:

- The oven temperature is set to 300 °F.
- Beat egg whites and cream of tartar until they have doubled in volume. After adding them, whip the mixture until firm peaks start to form.
- Use two teaspoons to transfer one tsp of meringue on a baking sheet covered with parchment paper. Use the back of the other spoon to do this
- After approximately 25 mins of baking at 300°F, the meringues ought to be crisp. Maintain in a sealed container.

Nutritional facts:

- Calories 37
- Fat: 0.9g
- Carbs: 9g
- Protein: 0.6g

10.7   Peachy pavlova

- Preparation time: 30 minutes
- Cooking time: 1 hour
- Serving: 8

Ingredients

- 4 (large) egg white
- ½ teaspoon vanilla extract
- 1 cup of sugar
- 2 cups peaches juice, canned
- ½ teaspoon cream tartar

Directions:

- Set the oven's temperature to 225°F.
- Put parchment paper on a baking pan and set it aside.
- The egg whites should be beaten for about a minute, or till soft peaks form, in a large bowl.
- Add cream of tartar by beating.
- The egg whites should be very stiff and shiny before you add the sugar, so add 1 tbsp. Do not overbeat.
- Blend in the vanilla.
- To create 8 rounds, evenly distribute the meringue on the baking sheet.
- In the center of each round, make an indentation with the bottom of the spoon.
- The meringues should be baked for about an hour or until a crusty, light brown layer appears.
- After turning off the oven, leave the meringues inside to cool overnight.
- Place the meringues on serving dishes after removing them from the sheet.
- Distribute the peaches evenly among the meringues' centers before serving.
- Meringues can be kept for up to a week at room

temperature in a sealed container

Nutritional facts:

- Calories 132
- Fat: 0g
- Carbs: 32g
- Protein: 2g

10.8 Pecan and raisin cookies (without sugar)

- Preparation time: 15 minutes
- Cooking time: 20 minutes
- Serving: 42 cookies

Ingredients

- 1 egg
- 1 ¾ cup flour
- ½ teaspoon salt
- ½ teaspoon cinnamon
- 2 teaspoon baking powder
- ½ teaspoon orange rind, grated
- ¼ cup oil
- ½ cup raisins
- ½ cup pecans
- ¾ cup orange juice, unsweetened

Directions:

- Cinnamon, salt, baking powder, and flour should all be combined.
- Add the remaining components.

- Mix well.
- Put teaspoonfuls at a time on an ungreased cookie sheet.
- Bake at 375 °F for 15 - 20 minutes.

Nutritional facts:

- Calories 60
- Fat: 4g
- Carbs: 6g
- Protein: 1g

10.9   <u>Cinnamon custard</u>

- Preparation time: 20 minutes
- Cooking time: 1 hour
- Serving: 6

Ingredients

- 4 eggs
- Butter, unsalted
- ¼ cup sugar, granulated
- ½ teaspoon cinnamon, ground
- 1 teaspoon vanilla extract
- 1½ cups of rice milk
- Cinnamon sticks for garnishing (optional)
    -
Directions:

The oven should be heated to 325°F.

- Place 6 (4-ounce) ramekins in a baking dish and lightly oil them; leave aside.
- In a large mixing bowl, thoroughly combine the rice milk,

sugar, eggs, cinnamon, and vanilla with a whisk.
- Through a fine strainer, pour the mixture into a pitcher.
- The custard should be evenly distributed among the ramekins.
- Hot water should be poured into the baking dish until it is halfway up the edges of the ramekins, being careful not to let any water spill into the ramekins themselves.
- Bake the custards for approximately one hour or until a knife inserted into the center of one custard comes out clean.
- The ramekins should be removed from the water, and the custards should be taken out of the oven.
- Once the custards have cooled for an hour on wire racks, they should be chilled for another hour in the fridge.
- If desired, add a cinnamon stick to the top of each custard.

Nutritional facts:
- Calories 110
- Fat: 4g
- Carbs: 14g
- Protein: 4g

10.10   Pound cake (Low sodium)
- Preparation time: 15 minutes
- Cooking time: 30 minutes
- Serving: 1/9 cake

Ingredients
- ¼ -pound butter, unsalted
- 1 ¼ cup of bread flour

- (large) eggs, beaten slightly
- ounces milk
- 3/4 cup of sugar

Directions:

- Add sugar gradually while you cream the butt; beat until fluffy.
- Add the milk, flour, and eggs.
- Mix well.
- With pan paper, line an 18x13-inch pan.
- Bake for 30 minutes at 375°F.

Nutritional facts:

- Calories 243
- Fat: 12g
- Carbs: 31g
- Protein: 3g

Bonus: 30 days meal plan

Days	Breakfast	Lunch	Dinner
1	Scrambled eggs with cheese and fresh herbs	Salad with strawberries and watercress with almond dressing	Seafood casserole
2	Loaded Vegetable Eggs	Soup with rotisserie chicken noodles	Beef barley soup with vegetables
3	Chai apple smoothie	Beef ginger salad	Herb-pesto tuna
4	Berry parfait	Soup with turkey bulgur	Pumpkin soup
5	Breakfast green soup	Cucumber-cilantro salsa with grilled steak	Grilled shrimp with a lime cucumber salsa
6	Apple-mint French toast	Kohlrabi soup	Sour and sweet meatloaf
7	Apple lemon smoothie	Fried rice with vegetables	Aromatic chicken and cabbage stir-fry
8	Morning herb rolls	Minestrone	Beef stir-up
9	Oat banana shake	Potato and cauliflower curry	Fettuccine with pork ragu
10	Leek and Brussels sprout quiche	Fish with pineapple salsa	Aromatic chicken and cabbage stir-fry
11	Chia pudding	Pumpkin soup	Cucumber-cilantro salsa with grilled steak
12	Raspberry peach smoothie	Salad of roasted beets	Kale and Salmon on parchment
13	Stuffed omelet with vegetables	Soup with a creamy vegetable mixture	Grilled shrimp with a lime cucumber salsa
14	Pina colada Smoothie	Shrimp scampi linguine	Garlic lemon halibut
15	Blueberry pancakes	Red pepper roasted soup	Mac and cheese

16	Egg and avocado bake	Delicious popcorn	Strata of red peppers
17	Kiwi watermelon smoothie	Chinese-style turkey salad	Vegetable Biryani
18	Asparagus frittata	Confetti farfalle salad	Seafood casserole
19	Corn pudding	Arugula and celery salad	Beef stir-up
20	Breakfast wrap with fruit and cheese	Cauliflower curried soup	Falafel spinach wrap
21	Breakfast burrito with green chilies	Lemon-dressed cucumber-dill salad with cabbage	Minestrone
22	Apple lemon smoothie	Spicy broccoli and tofu stir-fry	Bowl of roasted vegetables and barley
23	Buckwheat pancakes	Watercress and pear salad	Falafel spinach wrap
25	Raspberry peach smoothie	Thai-inspired vegetable curry	Kale and Salmon on parchment
26	Broccoli-basil quiche	Lemon-dressed cucumber-dill salad with cabbage	Soup with turkey bulgur
27	Chia vanilla smoothie	A butternut squash soup	Falafel spinach wrap
28	Berries mint water	Rice and collard-filled red peppers	Thai curried chicken
29	Hot multigrain cereal	Thai-inspired vegetable curry	Asian-style chicken satay
30	Mexican breakfast eggs on toast	Confetti farfalle salad	Cucumber-cilantro salsa with grilled steak

Printed in Great Britain
by Amazon

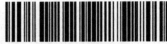